Felson's
principles of
Chest
Roentgenology

Felson's
principles of
Chest
Roentgen◆logy
a programmed text

Second Edition

LAWRENCE R. GOODMAN, M.D., F.A.C.R.
Professor of Radiology, Pulmonary Medicine and Intensive Care
Director, Thoracic Radiology
Medical College of Wisconsin
Milwaukee, Wisconsin

W.B. SAUNDERS COMPANY
A Division of Harcourt Brace and Company
Philadelphia ◆ London ◆ Toronto ◆ Montreal ◆ Sydney ◆ Tokyo

W.B. SAUNDERS COMPANY
A Division of Harcourt Brace & Company

The Curtis Center
Independence Square West
Philadelphia, Pennsylvania 19106

Library of Congress Cataloging-in-Publication Data

Goodman, Lawrence R. (Lawrence Roger).
Felson's principles of chest roentgenology: a programmed text.—2nd ed. / Lawrence R. Goodman.

p.   cm.

Rev. ed. of: Principles of chest roentgenology / Benjamin Felson . . . [et al.]. 1965.

ISBN 0–7216–7685–5

1. Chest—Radiography.   I. Felson, Benjamin.   II. Title.
[DNLM: 1. Radiography, Thoracic.   WF 975G653f 1999]

RC 941.G56   1999   617.5′407572—dc21

DNLM/DLC   98–36119

FELSON'S PRINCIPLES OF CHEST ROENTGENOLOGY:
A Programmed Text   ISBN 0–7216–7685–5

Printed in the United States of America.

Last digit is the print number: 9   8   7   6   5   4   3   2

This book is dedicated to my parents
Martha and Sidney Goodman
for years of support, encouragement, and love

Preface

Principles of Chest Roentgenology is one the best selling books in the history of radiology. It has been published in seven languages and is still selling, some 33 years after publication. Why has this unpretentious text been such an enduring success, despite the dramatic changes in medicine and imaging since initial publication? Drs. Felson, Weinstein, and Spitz were successful because the book is simple, relevant, interactive, repetitive, manageable, and fun.

Simple. The basic concepts are presented in a straightforward manner and logical sequence, one chapter building on the next.

Relevant. The text emphasizes basic radiographic anatomy and signs of disease seen in everyday practice. The chest x-ray is an important component in virtually every discipline in medicine.

Interactive. One cannot passively read this textbook. Active participation is engaging, entertaining, and the material is more likely to be remembered.

Repetitive, repetitive, repetitive. Important concepts are presented and re-presented from various points of view, reinforcing previously acquired knowledge.

Manageable. The open style and carefully selected material says to every harried reader, "This book is doable."

Fun. *Principles in Chest Roentgenology* proves that learning does not have to be tedious. It strikes a balance between serious purpose, important information, wit, and dialogue between the author and the reader. Many remember the jokes long after the details of left lower lobe anatomy have faded (probably not a terrible tragedy).

In the second edition, I have tried to retain the essence of *Fundamentals of Chest Radiology,* while updating the science. Computed tomography, ultrasound, and magnetic resonance imaging have been included to explain the conventional radiographic anatomy and to round out the imaging approach. Existing chapters have been updated and shortened. Five new chapters deal with cross-sectional imaging, an organized approach to reading the chest x-ray, and patterns of lung disease, mediastinal disease, and cardiac disease. All of the radiographs are new and their number increased.

The science is easy! The humor is difficult! Much of the joy of the original text is the quips and one-liners throughout the book. Some new material has been added and some material, no longer politically correct, has been deleted. Hopefully, the spirit of the book remains.

I have many people to thank for their help—Drs. Spitz and Weinstein and Mrs. Virginia Felson, Dr. Felson's equally witty and outgoing widow, for their encouragement while rewriting this book. Three colleagues in the Department of Radiology at the Medical College of Wisconsin, Drs. Ronald Kuzo, Christopher Griffin, and Daniel Malone have been gracious enough to review each chapter and to provide invaluable suggestions. The most helpful groups, however, have been the 1998 and 1999 Senior Classes of the Medical College of Wisconsin. While on their radiology elective, they have devoted many hours to critiquing the content, style, and grammar and correcting the speling. They were not shy!

This book was started while I was on sabbatical at the Policlinico at the University of Milan, Italy. To Professor Luciano Gattinoni and Dr. Emanuelle Fedrega, "grazie per l'aiuto e il sostegno."

Mrs. Sylvia Bartz, my senior administrative assistant, provided wonderful help from beginning to end. She provided e-mail, fax, and express mail support to Milan and outstanding secretarial support and good counsel in Milwaukee.

Writing a book, even a short one, is tremendously time-consuming. The patience and backing of a loving spouse is a great asset. Thank you, Hannah, for the encouragement and for providing the computer links between Milan and Milwaukee.

LAWRENCE R. GOODMAN, M.D.

Figure Credits

2–10	Dr. Andrew Taylor	Medical College of Wisconsin, Milwaukee, Wisconsin
2–11	Dr. Kiran Sagar	Medical College of Wisconsin, Milwaukee, Wisconsin
6–4	Dr. E. Martinez	Prescott, Arizona
7–3A	Ms. Ann Gorman	Medical College of Wisconsin, Milwaukee, Wisconsin
11–9 and 11–16	Dr. Sanford Rubin	University of Texas, Galveston, Texas
11–4D	Dr. Francisco Quiroz	Medical College of Wisconsin, Milwaukee, Wisconsin
12–11	The late Dr. Wylie Dodds	Medical College of Wisconsin, Milwaukee, Wisconsin
12–13	Dr. Emanuelle Fedrega	Universita' delgi Studi di Milano, Milan, Italy
Q–4	Dr. Jack Sty	Children's Hospital of Wisconsin, Milwaukeé, Wisconsin
Q–9	Dr. Timothy Klostermeier	Wilmington, Ohio

Thanks to Mr. Stanton Himelhoch (photographer) and Mr. Robert Fenn (illustrator) of Medical Center Graphics, Milwaukee, Wisconsin.

⸺ *Instructions* ⸺◆

Most of you are familiar with programmed learning. The numbered frames on the left side of each page require a response. Questions are designed, in most instances, to help you make the correct response: The answer is often made clear by the frame itself or what you have learned in earlier frames. In those frames that offer multiple choices, merely circle the one or more correct answers. When there are blanks, fill in the answer. The answer to each frame will be found on the right side of the page and appropriately numbered. Use the mask, in the back of the book, to hide the answers to the frame. We prefer you write your answers in ink so that your friends will have to buy their own copies.

It is not essential that your answers be identical to ours, as long as the meaning is the same. If you miss an answer, reread the frame so that you will be better prepared for what is to come. It is okay to cheat by looking at the answers first, since it's your money and time. Since your concentrated attention is required, we suggest that you set a limit of an hour, at most, of consecutive study.

At the end of each chapter is a Review Section summarizing the most important concepts. Don't skip them. "Ten Great Cases," the quiz that follows the last chapter, contains carefully selected x-rays that allow you to synthesize and apply your new knowledge. If you don't do well, blame us.

I hope our attempts at humor and informality make the learning process pleasant and relaxing. Before going to Chapter 1, try the samples below.

1. This text is based on the reader's participation.	*1.*
a. Mark Twain once said, "It is better to keep your mouth shut and appear [stupid/smart] than to open it and _____."	*a. stupid* *remove all doubt*
b. Lee Rogers, M.D. once said, "Don't let the fear of being [right/wrong] interfere with the joy of being _____.	*b. wrong* *right*
c. We expect you to adopt philosophy [a./b.].	*c. b.*

2. Understanding the anatomy and the radiographic signs are the keys to reading x-rays.

   a. "You'd be surprised how much you observe by _____," said Lawrence (Yogi) Berra.

   b. "You only see what you _____," says Lawrence R. Goodman, M.D.

   c. This book was written based on assumption [a./b.].

2.

a. watching

b. know

c. b.

Contents

The Radiographic Examination

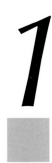

1

The chest x-ray is part of every physician's practice. He/she should have a basic understanding of the anatomy and pathology visible on the radiograph. In just 12 short, interactive (and occasionally humorous) chapters, you will learn a systematic approach to reading the x-ray, the normal anatomy of the lungs, and the basic patterns of lung disease.

1

Let's start with the standard frontal view of the chest, the posteroanterior radiograph, or the "PA chest." The term posteroanterior refers to the direction of the x-ray beam, which in this case traverses the patient from _____ to _____ .

1

posterior/anterior

2

By convention, the routine frontal view is taken with the patient upright and in full inspiration. The x-ray beam is horizontal and the x-ray tube is 6 feet from the film. This is what you get when you order a _____ view.

2

posteroanterior or "PA chest"

3

The PA view is taken at a distance of _____ feet to reduce magnification and enhance sharpness. Placing the part to be x-rayed close to the x-ray cassette (film) also reduces magnification and increases sharpness. See for yourself: Place your hand, palm down, 3 or 4 inches from a desktop, under a desk lamp (bulb type) or a flashlight. Observe the shadow.

(a) Flex your middle finger only. Its shadow gets [wider/narrower] and appears [sharper/less sharp]. That finger also appears foreshortened.

(b) If the light source (i.e., x-ray tube) moves further away, magnification [increases/decreases] and the margins become [sharper/less sharp].

3
six

(a) *narrower (less magnification)/sharper*

(b) *decreases sharper*

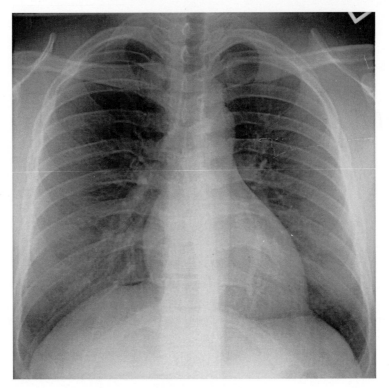

Figure 1–1A

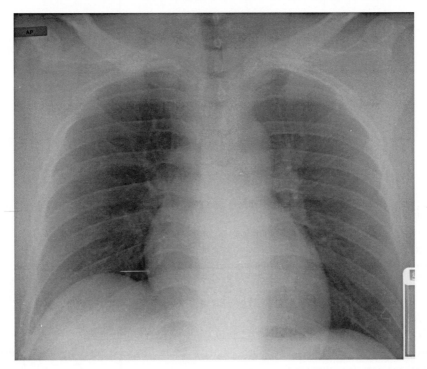

Figure 1–1B

4

To reduce the magnification and increase image sharpness, the chest should be as [close to/far from] the x-ray cassette as possible and the x-ray tube as [close to/far from] the cassette as practical.

4

close to
far from

5

The anteroposterior (AP) view, on the other hand, is usually made with a portable x-ray unit on very sick patients, who are unable to stand, and on infants. The patient is supine or sitting in bed. In this instance, the x-ray beam passes through the patient from _____ to _____ .

5

anterior
posterior

The AP view is taken supine or sitting rather than prone because it is less awkward for the sick patient and the infant usually squawks less when he/she can see what's happening.

6

Because portable x-ray units are less powerful than regular units, and because space is tight at the bedside, AP views are usually taken at shorter distances from the film. Compared with the PA radiograph, the AP radiograph has [greater/less] magnification and [more/less] sharp images. (If you missed this answer you should repeat the experiment in Frame 3.)

6

greater/less

The PA upright is preferred to the AP supine view because 1) there is less magnification and the image is sharper; 2) the erect patient inspires more deeply, showing more lung; and 3) pleural air and fluid are easier to see on the erect film.

7

Figure 1–1A and B are two films of the same patient, one AP and one PA. Which is the PA? _____ How did you decide? _____

7

Figure 1–1A is the PA
Sharper, less magnification, deeper inspiration

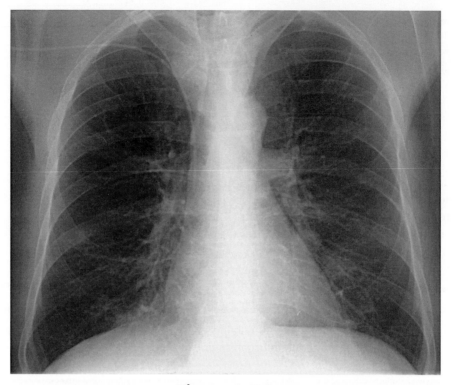

Figure 1–2A

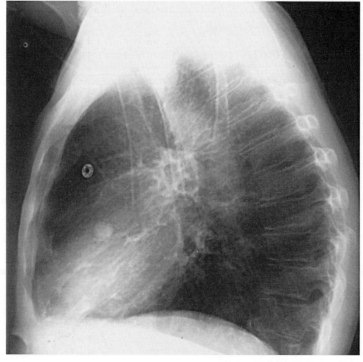

Figure 1–2B

Frontal radiographs, AP or PA, are viewed as if you were facing the patient. In Figure 1–2A, and in all x-rays, the patient's left is to your right.

8

The other routine view is the lateral. By convention, the left side of the chest is held against the x-ray cassette. This is called a _____ view. Like the PA view, it is also taken at _____ feet.

left lateral
six

If we were consistent, we would call it a right–left lateral, but "a foolish consistency is the hobgoblin of little minds" (Emerson). We just call it a lateral view.

9

It is common for a lesion located behind the heart, the mediastinum, or the diaphragm to be invisible on the PA view. The _____ view will generally show such a lesion, so we use it routinely.

lateral

Figure 1–2A and B. The nodule, superimposed on the heart, is easily seen on the lateral view. On the frontal (PA) view, it is hard to see along the left heart border. (Figure 1–2B, metallic artifact = pajama snap.)

10

On the lateral, which is routinely taken with the [right/left] side against the cassette, a right-sided nodule will appear [larger/smaller] than an identical left-sided nodule.

left
larger

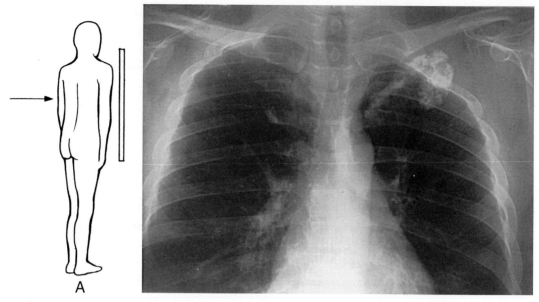

Figure 1–3A

Figure 1–3B

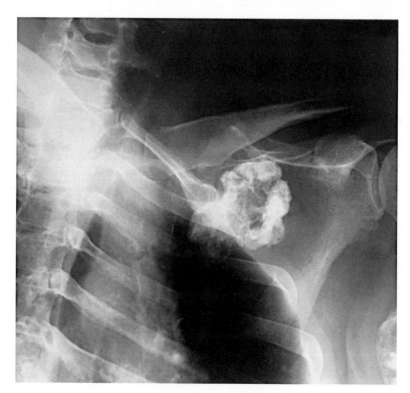

Figure 1–3C

11

In Figure 1–3*A,* the patient is in the right anterior oblique position. His (left/right) chest is against the cassette and the radiograph is taken in the PA direction.

11

right

12

When a patient turns from the straight PA to the right anterior oblique position, different anatomic structures move in different directions. In the right anterior oblique, the left pectoralis muscle or breast (anterior structures) move (medially/laterally), and the left scapula (a posterior structure) moves (medially/laterally), relative to the thorax. The opposite, of course, occurs in the left anterior oblique.

12

laterally
medially

13

Oblique views can help us localize lesions and eliminate superimposed structures. Figure 1–3*B* is a PA radiograph, showing a calcified mass over the upper thorax on the (left/right). In Figure 1–3*C,* in the right anterior oblique, the mass moves (medially/laterally), relative to the thorax. It must be located (anteriorly/posteriorly).

13

left
laterally
anteriorly

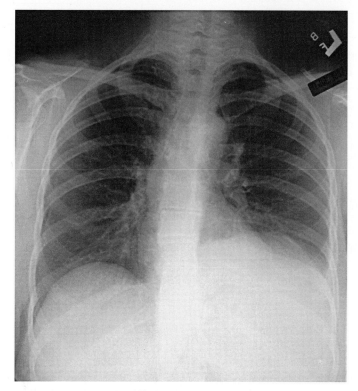

Figure 1–4A

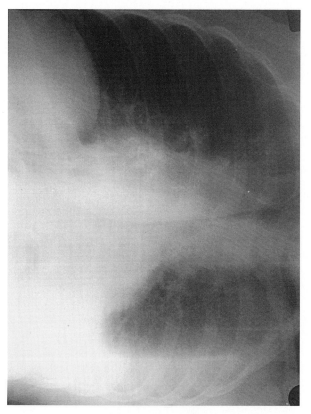

Figure 1–4B

14

What other views are there? Free fluid in the pleural cavity is affected by gravity. Fluid will gravitate toward the diaphragm when the patient is [erect/supine], toward the back when the patient is [erect/supine], and toward the lateral aspect of the dependent thorax when the patient lies on his or her _____ in the *lateral decubitus position.* (Decubitus = lying down. Lateral decubitus = lying on the side. [I looked it up].)

14

erect

supine

side

In Figure 1–4A, an upright film, what appears to be an elevated left hemidiaphragm is really free pleural fluid that has gravitated to the bottom of the left pleural space. This is confirmed in Figure 1–4B, made with the patient lying left side down (left lateral decubitus position). The fluid now layers against the dependent thoracic wall. This radiograph is obtained with a horizontal x-ray beam, i.e., parallel to the bed or x-ray table.

Sign in Doctor's Office: Everyone brings JOY to this office, some when they enter and some when they leave.

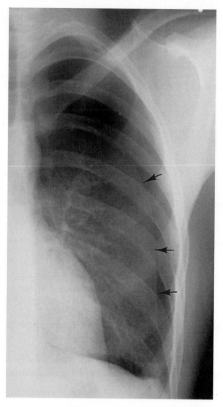

Figure 1–5

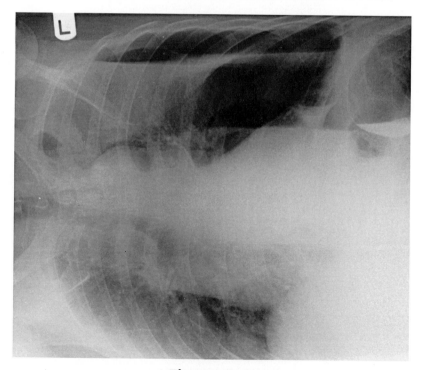

Figure 1–6

15

While intrapleural fluid falls with gravity, intrapleural air _____ . Therefore, the ideal position to diagnose a pneumothorax (intrapleural air) is [erect/supine]. If you suspect a left pneumothorax in a patient who can't stand or sit, a lateral decubitus film with the [left/right] side down is helpful. This is called the _____ position.

15

rises
erect

right
right lateral decubitus

Figure 1–5 shows a pneumothorax in the erect position (arrows delineate edge of lung). Figure 1–6 shows air between the lung and the left chest wall in the right lateral decubitus position.

16

The normal chest film is made on [inspiration/expiration]. On expiration, the lung markings become more crowded. There is less air in the lung, so the lung appears [whiter/blacker]. The heart, which sits on the diaphragm, is elevated and appears [larger/smaller].

16

inspiration

whiter

larger

Clinical Pearl: Caution, the supine or sitting patient often cannot inspire deeply. Therefore, many portable radiographs are not at full inspiration and may *simulate* disease.

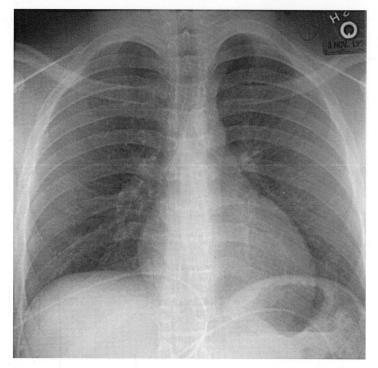

Figure 1–7A

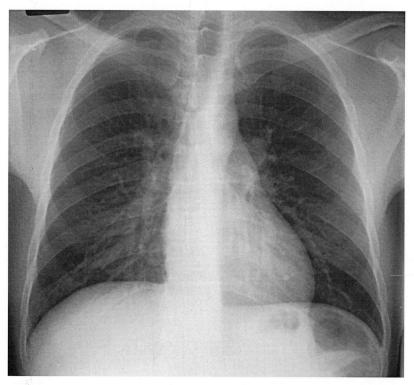

Figure 1–7B

A favorite trick of radiologists is to test a student with a normal *expiratory* radiograph. Figure 1–7A suggests cardiac enlargement and perhaps mild edema. Figure 1–7B was made on inspiration a few hours later and is normal.

17

Expiratory films can be used to one's advantage. An expiratory film can be used to detect focal air trapping from asymmetrical emphysema or a partial bronchial obstruction that impedes air flow on expiration (air trapping). Since the air in the obstructed lung cannot be expelled readily, that lung (or lobe) remains [inflated/deflated] on expiration while the the the rest of lung _____ , normally.

17

inflated
deflates

18

With unilateral air trapping, the normal deflated lung will appear [whiter/blacker/unchanged] while the obstructed lung will appear [whiter/blacker/unchanged].

18

whiter
unchanged

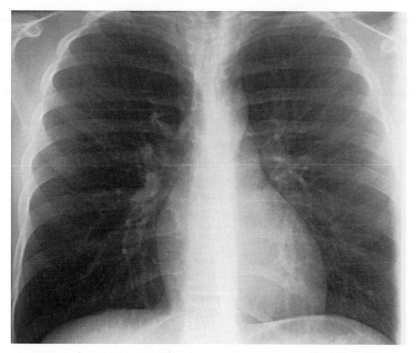

Figure 1–8A

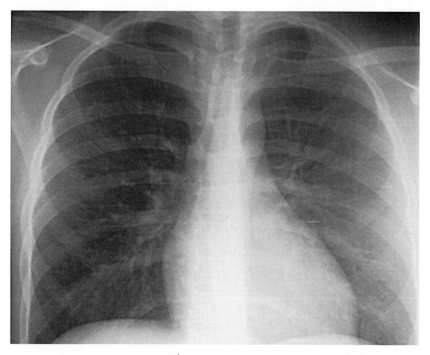

Figure 1–8B

In Figure 1–8A, the right lung is slightly blacker than the left lung. In Figure 1–8B, an expiratory film, the left deflates normally and gets whiter, while the right remains inflated and black. This was due to air trapping behind an aspirated foreign body.

Clinical Pearl: If you hear a unilateral wheeze, order an expiratory film to look for air trapping.

19

An expiratory x-ray may accentuate a small pneumothorax. On expiration, the deflated lung appears [whiter/blacker] compared with the intrapleural air and the fixed amount of intrapleural air is relatively [larger/smaller] in the smaller hemithorax.

19

whiter

larger

Logical? Yes! Helpful? Seldom! This technique is overrated but many still order it. Will you?

20

The expiratory radiograph is a two-edged sword. It simulates disease when decreased aeration causes the lung to appear [lighter/darker] and the elevated heart appears [bigger/smaller/unchanged]. Conversely, it is very helpful in the diagnosis of _____ and rarely helpful in the diagnosis of _____ .

20

lighter
bigger
focal air trapping
pneumothorax

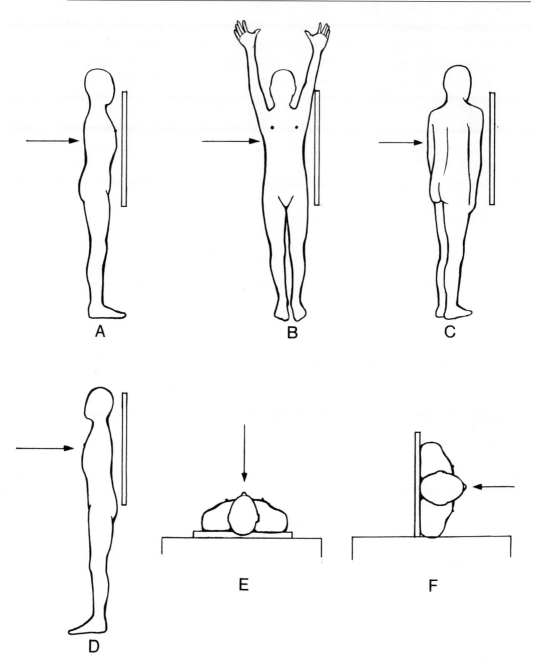

Figure 1–9

21

Let's review the various radiographic positions. What views are illustrated in Figure 1–9A–F?

A. _____   D. _____
B. _____   E. _____
C. _____   F. _____

21

A. PA
B. lateral (left)
C. right anterior oblique
D. AP
E. AP supine
F. right lateral decubitus

Two older techniques, the apical lordotic position and tomography (laminography), were used to display areas obscured by overlapping structures. The apical lordotic radiograph is a frontal view taken with the x-ray beam angled to project the clavicles above the lung apex to display disease hidden behind the clavicles. Tomography is a complex technique that utilizes an x-ray tube and cassette that move in opposite directions, keeping *only* the level of interest in focus. Both techniques have been largely replaced by better quality chest radiographs and computed tomography (CT)—two fewer things you have to learn!

22

All techniques discussed thus far produce static images—a subsecond snapshot of the thorax. Fluoroscopy, which is real-time x-ray viewed on a video monitor, provides information about moving organs. Examples include motion of the _____ during respiration and left ventricular _____ during systole. During fluoroscopy, the patient can be turned obliquely, to eliminate _____ of structures.

22

diaphragm or chest wall
contraction
overlapping
(superimposition)

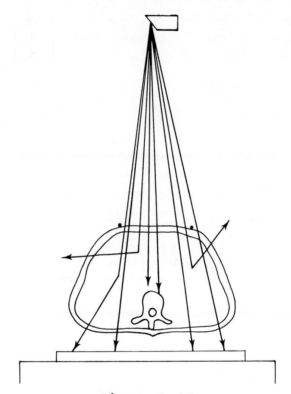

Figure 1–10

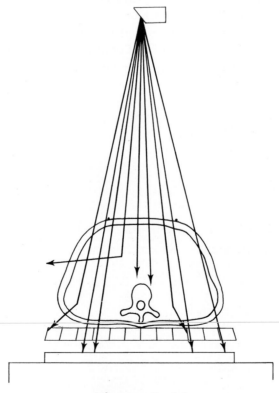

Figure 1–11

Let's finish with a few technical points. What causes the blacks, whites, and grays of an x-ray image? The x-ray beam contains x-ray photons of differing energies. As the x-ray photons pass through the patient, some are absorbed completely, some penetrate directly to the x-ray film, and some are deflected (scattered). Some of the scattered photons continue toward the x-ray film (Fig. 1–10).

23

Differential absorption and penetration of the x-ray photons create the x-ray image. [Direct/scattered] radiation exposes the film randomly, causing a background fog (loss of contrast), rather than useful information. In Figure 1–10, the image is formed by _____ x-rays and degraded by _____ x-rays.

23

scattered
(deflected)

direct
scattered

The differential absorption of radiation by different tissues or diseases is responsible for all radiographic images. Air, fat, soft tissue (muscle, fluid), and bone absorb progressively more radiation.

24

Bone absorbs [more/less] radiation and air absorbs [more/less] radiation. Bone is said to be radiodense, because radiation [hardly/easily] penetrates it. The lung is deemed radiolucent because radiation [hardly/easily] penetrates it. (Absorption = 1/penetration.)

24

more
less
hardly
easily

25

Scattered radiation [increases/decreases] contrast, degrading the image. A grid can be used to absorb scattered radiation before it hits the film. A grid is a large thin plate composed of very thin parallel strips of lead and wood. As shown in Figure 1–11, the wood strips permit most of the [direct/scattered] x-rays to reach the film, while the lead strips absorb many of the [direct/scattered] photons.

25

decreases

direct
scattered

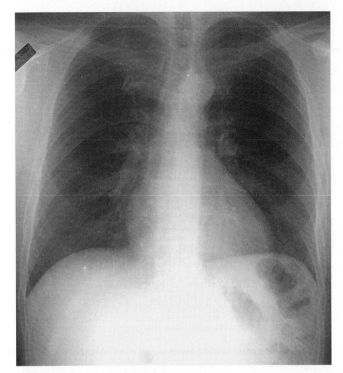

Figure 1–12A

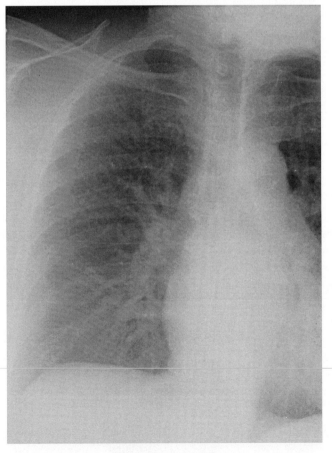

Figure 1–12B

26

The grid reduces _____ but leaves annoying "lead absorption lines (grid lines)." Moving the grid during the x-ray exposure [sharpens/blurs] these lines, minimizing the "grid artifact". The moving grid is called a "Bucky grid" after [Gustav Bucky, its founder/Bucky Badger, the University of Wisconsin mascot].

26

scattered radiation

blurs

Gustav Bucky

27

In Figure 1–12*A* and *B*, which of the chest radiographs was taken with a grid? _____ How did you know? _____

27

Figure 1–12A

Better contrast, sharper image

What causes the x-ray film to be black or white? An unexposed x-ray film is housed in a lightproof cassette, sandwiched between two phosphorescent screens. X-rays hit the phosphorescent screens, the screens give off light, and the light exposes the film. Heavy exposure (e.g., through radiolucent lung) precipitates much silver, which causes the film to be black. Little light exposure (e.g., through radiodense bone) precipitates little silver, which causes the film to be white. (More technical stuff in Chapter 6—try to resist peeking.)

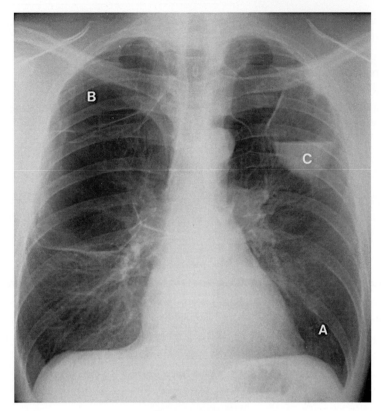

Figure 1–13

REVIEW

I

For the sharpest, truest images, the patient should be as [close to/far from] the cassette as possible. The x-ray tube should be [4 ft/5 ft/6 ft] from the cassette. The effects of scattered radiation are minimized with a _____ .

I

close to
6 ft
grid (Bucky grid)

II

Which view or technique, other than the routine PA and lateral, would give the most information in the following situations?
(a) free pleural fluid on the right: _____
(b) suspected air trapping behind an endobronchial tumor: _____
(c) suspected right pneumothorax in patient who can't sit or stand: _____
(d) bullet fragment, possibly in heart: _____
(e) nodule, possibly in lung or in rib: _____

II

(a) right lateral decubitus

(b) expiratory

(c) left lateral decubitus

(d) fluoroscopy
(e) oblique or fluoroscopy

III

(a) In emphysema, excess _____ is trapped in the lung. The air [absorbs/transmits] most radiation, which stimulates the [cassette/screen] to produce light. The x-ray film appears excessively [dark/light] in the emphysematous regions.
(b) Fluid (effusion, blood, pus) is more radiodense. It absorbs [less/more] radiation than a normal lung. The diseased area appears [dark/light].
(c) In Figure 1–13, area _____ is through normal radiolucent lung, area _____ is through hyperlucent lung (emphysema, bulla), and area _____ is through radiodense lung (fluid in a bulla).

III
(a) air
    transmits
    screen
    dark

(b) more
    light
(c) A = normal
    B = hyperlucent
    C = radiodense

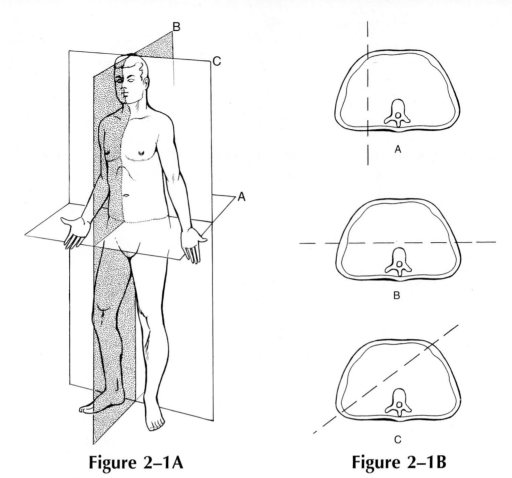

Figure 2–1A

Figure 2–1B

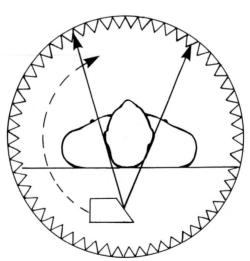

Figure 2–2

Cross-Sectional Imaging Techniques

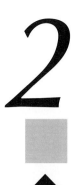

Three relatively recent imaging techniques, computed tomography (CT), ultrasound (US), and magnetic resonance imaging (MRI), have greatly improved thoracic imaging. In all conventional x-ray techniques, the x-ray beam passes through the patient, superimposing all structures in its path onto an x-ray film (projection image). Cross-sectional scanning techniques "slice" the patient open, providing a look "inside," eliminating superimposition. These images are the product of multiple digital readings, from multiple angles, synthesized by a computer into a digital image. Digital imaging data can be processed to improve tissue contrast or change image orientation. Even conventional radiographs can now be done using a digital receptor in place of film.

1

All cross-sectional imaging can be viewed in the "axial, sagittal, coronal, or oblique planes."

(a) An image perpendicular to the long axis of the patient is a(n) _____ image.

(b) An image parallel to the lateral plane is a(n) _____ image.

(c) An image parallel to the patient's frontal plane is a(n) _____ image.

(d) All other images are _____ images.

1

(a) axial

(b) sagittal

(c) coronal

(d) oblique

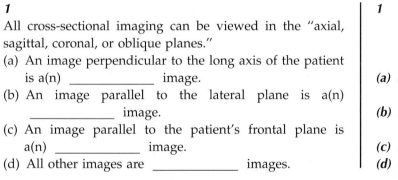

Figure 2–1*A* demonstrates the axial (A), sagittal (B), and coronal (C) planes. Figure 2–1*B* demonstrates the relationship of the sagittal (A), coronal (B), and oblique (C) planes to the axial plane.

CT provides the most useful cross-sectional imaging of the chest. The patient is on a mobile table that passes through a cylindrical tunnel or gantry. In the gantry wall, an x-ray tube revolves around the patient (Fig. 2–2). The x-ray beam hits multiple detectors in the opposite gantry wall. The radiation is quantified and synthesized into a digital image. (Don't ask how—it's quite complicated.)

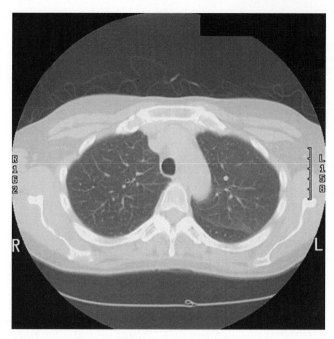

Figure 2–3A

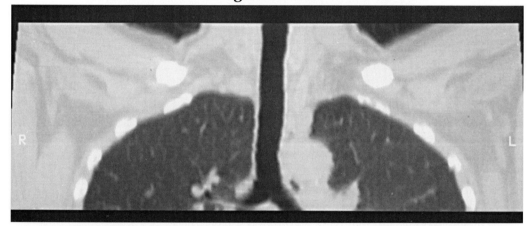

Figure 2–3B

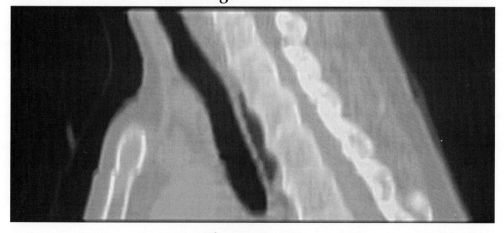

Figure 2–3C

2

The CT scanner routinely produces a(n) [axial/coronal/sagittal] image (Fig. 2–3*A*). In Figure 2–3*B*, the same data set is reconstructed in the _____ plane of the trachea. In Figure 2–3*C*, it is through the _____ plane of the trachea.

| *2* |
| *axial* |
| *coronal* |
| *sagittal* |

The same digital data, in memory, can be sampled in subsets to optimize the contrast for each type of tissue. In the thorax, it is routine to look at images reconstructed to show lung detail ("lung window") and reconstructed to show mediastinal detail ("soft tissue or mediastinal window").

3

Figure 2–3*A* is a(n) [axial/sagittal/coronal] image reconstructed to show [lung/mediastinal] detail, while Figure 2–4 shows [lung/mediastinal] detail in the same patient. To achieve this, the patient was scanned [twice/once].

| *3* |
| *axial* |
| *lung* |
| *mediastinal* |
| *once* |

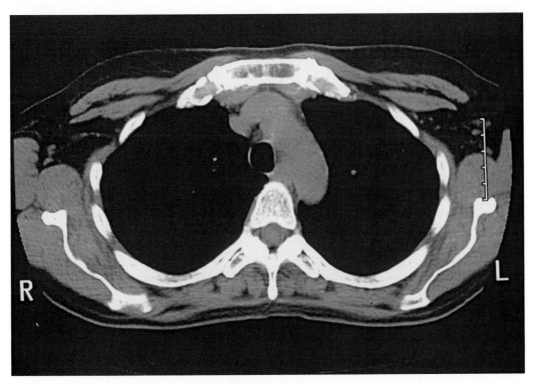

Figure 2–4

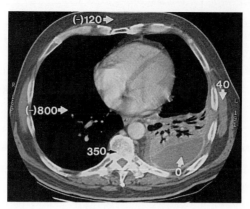

Figure 2–5

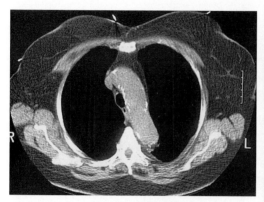

Figure 2–6A

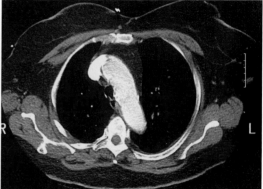

Figure 2–6B

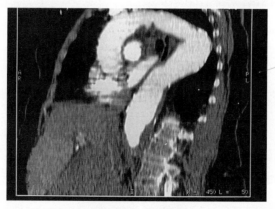

Figure 2–6C

4

Both radiography and CT utilize x-rays. By convention, the synthesized CT image of the normal lung is black because the lung is radio _____ . The bone is white because it is radio _____ . Muscle, water, and fat absorb progressively less radiation and are progressively [lighter/darker] shades of gray.

4

lucent

dense

darker

5

Conventional radiographs are able to distinguish four basic tissue densities. In order of increasing absorption, they are:

(a) _____ (c) _____

(b) _____ (d) _____

5

(a) air
(b) fat
(c) soft tissue (water)
(d) bone (metal)

CT has better contrast discrimination and easily distinguishes among muscle, fluid (blood, bile, etc.), and fat. CT density is expressed in Hounsfield units (HUs). The scanner is calibrated so that pure water = 0 HU. Typical HU values are: lung = (−)800, fat = (−)120, fluid = 0, muscle = 40, and bone = 350. Figure 2–5 demonstrates the various CT densities in HUs.

6

Although [x-ray/CT] has better contrast discrimination, the heart, the vessels, the mediastinal structures, and the muscles are similar intermediate shades of gray. This soft tissue density is approximately [−40/0/40] HU. Iodinated contrast is often given intravenously during the scan to increase the radiodensity of blood. The heart and vessels then absorb [more/less] radiation than surrounding structures and appear [white/black].

6

CT

40

more
white

Figure 2–6A is an axial CT scan emphasizing the soft tissue or mediastinal structures ("mediastinal or soft tissue windows"). In Figure 2–6B, intravenous contrast was given during scanning. Note the change in the density of the aortic arch and the superior vena cava. Figure 2–6C is a left anterior oblique reconstruction, using the same digital data, to evaluate the aneurysmal proximal descending aorta.

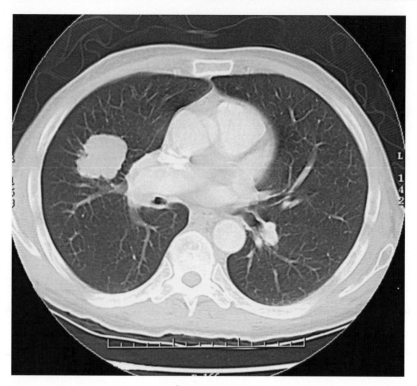

Figure 2–7

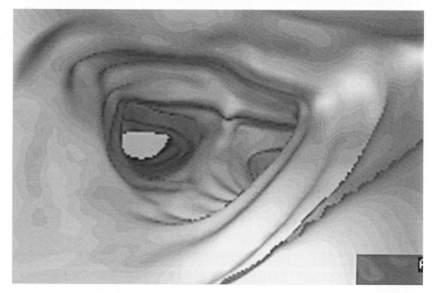

Figure 2–8

7

Axial images assume you are viewing the patient from below (looking up from the feet). The patient's right is on your left (as in the chest x-ray). In Figure 2–7, the _____ lung is normal. The branching structures that taper peripherally are the _____ . The radiolucent areas are the air-containing lung parenchyma. The right lung contains a tumor. It absorbs _____ radiation than normal lungs. The tumor is radio _____ .

7

left
pulmonary vessels

more
dense

8

More powerful computers create more powerful images. They create 3-dimensional images that can be viewed from any direction. The same data set used for Figure 2–3 provides a 3-dimensional view of the _____ in Figure 2–8. This is virtual bronchoscopy.

8

trachea (carina)

Magnetic resonance imaging (MRI) uses magnetic fields rather than radiation to form an image. To oversimplify, the patient is exposed in a gantry to a high-intensity magnetic field and a brief radiofrequency (RF) pulse. The various tissue components (water, fat, etc.) are excited differently by the RF pulse. When the RF pulse ends, the perturbed tissues return to their resting state, releasing energy, which is quantitated and synthesized into a digital image. MRI is very flexible. Unlike that of x-ray and CT images, the imaging gray scale varies greatly with the applied radiofrequency pulses. (These are too varied to describe here but they do provide employment for thousands of imaging physicists.) Unfortunately, because lung (air) and bone give little signal, MRI is of limited use in the thorax. MRI is especially good for fluid-containing structures, like the heart and vessels, and for solid masses. MRI is expensive and cumbersome and is used most often to evaluate some cardiovascular and some mediastinal problems.

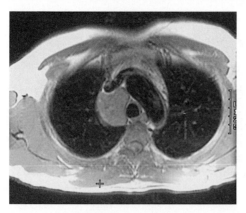

Figure 2–9A

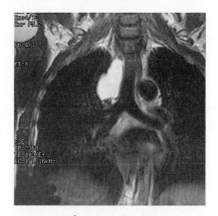

Figure 2–9B

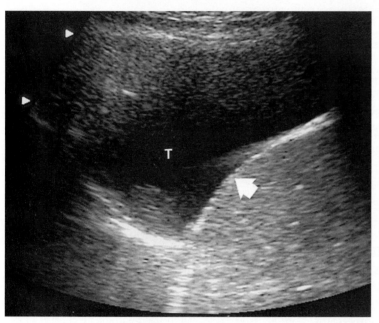

Figure 2–10A

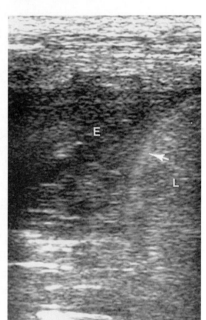

Figure 2–10B

9

The gray scale (blacks, whites, and grays) of MRI [does/ does not] correspond to the densities of x-ray images. One would have to know which _____ was used in order to understand the gray scale.

9

does not
radiofrequency pulse

Figure 2–9 shows two MRI sequences of the same patient, with a right middle mediastinal mass. In the axial image, Figure 2–9A, the paratracheal mass is gray. In the coronal image, Figure 2–9B, the paratracheal mass is white. The varying responses to the RF pulses help MRI to characterize tissue.

In ultrasound (US) or sonography, a transducer directs high-frequency sound waves into the body, much the way the Navy uses sonar. The sound waves reflect differently off different tissues. The transducer then detects reflected sound waves and a computer synthesizes them into diagnostic images. Fluid causes minimal reflection so it appears as a homogeneous low-signal area (low echogenicity). Soft tissue absorbs, reflects, and deflects, causing a heterogeneous echogenic area. Sound waves travel poorly in air and bone. Bone/soft tissue and air/soft tissue interfaces are hyperreflective. Therefore, air-filled lung and bone are very difficult to evaluate with ultrasound. US is relatively inexpensive, portable, and especially suited for imaging pleural or pericardial fluid and cardiovascular structures.

10

Ultrasound is particularly valuable for evaluating [pneumothorax/empyema]. A simple pleural effusion (transudate) shows a low and [heterogeneous/homogeneous] signal. An empyema appears [heterogeneous/homogeneous].

10

empyema
homogeneous
heterogeneous

Figure 2–10 shows two sagittal ultrasounds through the right pleural space. Figure 2–10A is a hypoechoic pleural transudate (T). Figure 2–10B is a hyperechoic exudate (E). (L = liver; arrow = diaphragm.)

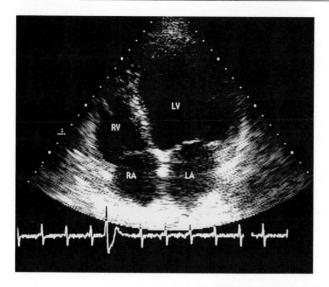

Figure 2–11

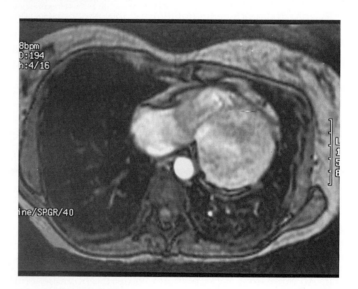

Figure 2–12A

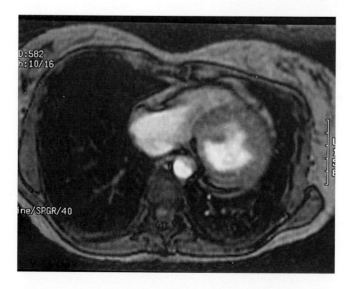

Figure 2–12B

Both MRI and ultrasound are capable of very rapid repetitive image acquisition. This permits evaluation of some dynamic physiological processes such as cardiac motion and blood flow. Figure 2–11, an echocardiogram (ultrasound), demonstrates the four cardiac chambers. Figure 2–12A and B, MRI images, show the left ventricle in diastole and systole.

11

Match the clinical problem with the *best* imaging modality:

A—pleural effusion _____   1—MRI

B—emphysema _____   2—US

C—cardiac function _____   3—neither

D—rib fracture _____   4—both

E—tumor invading
　　mediastinum _____

11

A = 2

B = 3

C = 4

D = 3

E = 1

Now that you are in medicine, it is certain that at some family gathering, Aunt Rose will ask you, "Exactly how safe is x-ray?" As with most important things, there are no simple answers. Diagnostic levels of radiation are generally considered safe for the individual, with the potential diagnostic benefits outweighing the barely measurable, but real, population risks associated with diagnostic levels of ionizing radiation. The major risks are genetic damage and potential cancer induction. Conventional chest radiographs produce *very, very low* radiation exposure, whereas studies such as CT, fluoroscopy, and angiography give considerably higher doses. Radiation dose is cumulative over a lifetime (unlike an old love affair, it doesn't "wear off" with time). Therefore, patient radiation dose should be kept to a minimum. This is especially true during the reproductive years, during pregnancy, and during childhood, because rapidly dividing cells are more sensitive to radiation damage. The best way to reduce patient exposure is to *choose the correct imaging examination.* If you are unsure, discuss it with the radiologist.

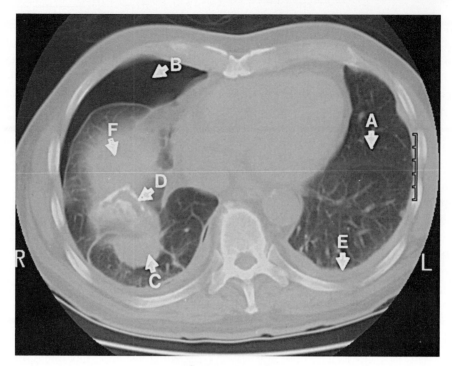

Figure 2–13

REVIEW

I

Conventional radiographs distinguish four basic tissue densities. They are _____ , _____ , _____ , and _____ . [CT scans/radiographs] have better contrast discrimination.

II

The ultrasound of a pericardial effusion (transudate) would be expected to be [homogeneous/heterogeneous] and have [low/high] echogenicity, whereas loculated pericardial infection would be [homogeneous/heterogeneous] and of [low/high] echogenicity.

III

The CT in Figure 2–13 shows multiple intrathoracic densities. Match the areas with their approximate Hounsfield values:

A—normal left lung _____   (+)350 HU
B—pneumothorax _____   (+)40 HU
C—lung mass _____   0 HU
D—calcified diaphragm _____ (−)800 HU
E—pleural effusion _____   (−)1000 HU
F—dome of diaphragm _____

IV

Diagnostic radiation should be held to a minimum in (check one or more):
(a)   children
(b)   cancer patients
(c)   pregnant women
(d)   lawyers

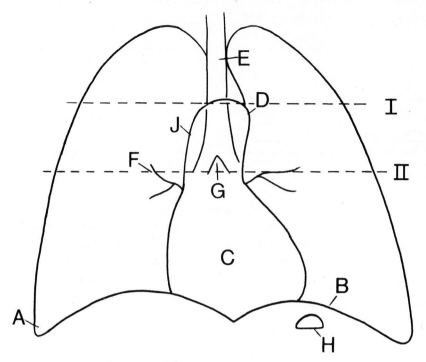

Figure 3–1A

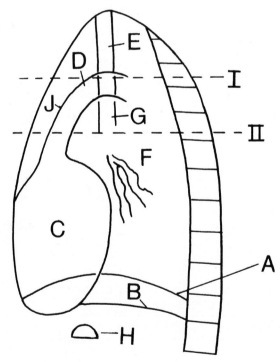

Figure 3–1B

The Normal Chest X-Ray: Reading Like the Pros

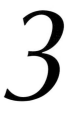

3

The keys to reading x-rays well are a good understanding of normal anatomy and an orderly search pattern. This chapter will reacquaint you with the normal anatomy and then develop a search pattern that you can apply to every film. By being systematic, you will miss fewer important findings. Not that experienced hands don't miss findings; they just miss fewer findings. Learn this ordered approach and then stick to it—*film after film.* You will look like a pro.

1

If you put the film on the view box backward, you will look like a [pro/turkey]. A PA or an AP film is always hung as if you are facing the patient from the [front/back].

2

You already know most of the anatomy; you just haven't thought about it in terms of a PA and a lateral projection. Remember, these are projection images, so all anatomic structures in the x-ray beam are _____ . Mentally, you must fuse two projection images into a 3-dimensional image.

3

Test yourself on Figure 3–1*A* and *B*. Study these diagrams until you could give these answers in your sleep (perhaps you are already doing that).

Posterior/Anterior

A. _____   D. _____   G. _____
B. _____   E. _____   H. _____
C. _____   F. _____   J. _____

Lateral

A. _____   D. _____   G. _____
B. _____   E. _____   H. _____
C. _____   F. _____   J. _____

1

front

2

superimposed

3

A. *costophrenic sulcus (angle)*
B. *left diaphragm*
C. *heart*
D. *aortic knob (arch)*
E. *trachea*
F. *hilum*
G. *carina*
H. *stomach bubble*
J. *ascending aorta*

39

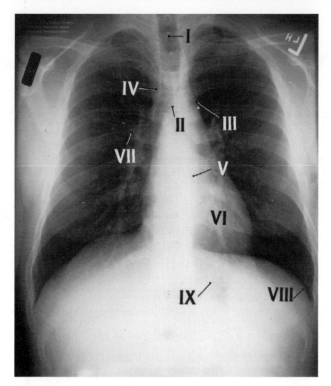

Figure 3–2A

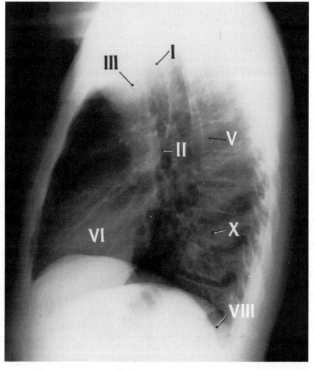

Figure 3–2B

4

Label radiographs in Figure 3–2*A* and *B*.

PA Radiograph

I	_____	VI	_____
II	_____	VII	_____
III	_____	VIII	_____
IV	_____	IX	_____
V	_____		

Lateral Radiograph

I	_____	VI	_____
II	_____	VIII	_____
III	_____	X	_____
V	_____		

4

I. **trachea**

II. **carina**

III. **aortic knob**

IV. **ascending aorta**

V. **descending aorta**

VI. **heart**

VII. **hilum**

VIII. **costophrenic sulcus (angle)**

IX. **stomach bubble**

X. **spine**

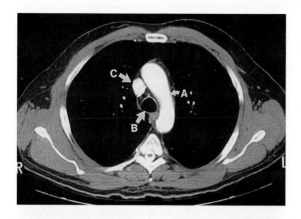

Figure 3–3A

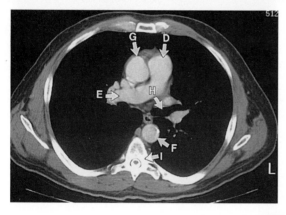

Figure 3–3B

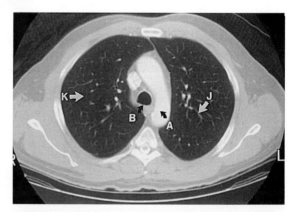

Figure 3–4A

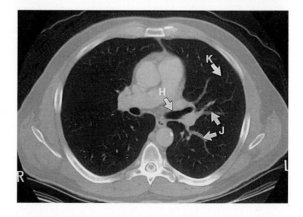

Figure 3–4B

You are now ready to tackle CT's. Use your knowledge of radiographic anatomy to understand the CT anatomy. The CT anatomy will then help you understand the anatomic relationships on the x-ray. Figure 3–3A and B are at mediastinal (soft tissue) windows and Figure 3–4A and B are at lung windows.

5

Figure 3–3A and B are photographed at _____ windows. Figure 3–3A corresponds to level I in Figure 3–1 and Figure 3–3B corresponds to level II in Figure 3–1. Identify:

A. _____ F. _____
B. _____ G. _____
C. _____ H. _____
D. _____ I. _____
E. _____

5

mediastinal (soft tissue)
A. aortic arch
B. trachea
C. superior vena cava
D. main pulmonary artery (Pulm trunk)
E. right pulmonary artery
F. descending aorta
G. ascending aorta
H. left main bronchus
I. vertebral body

6

In Figure 3–4A and B, photographed at _____ windows, identify:

A. _____ J. _____
B. _____ K. _____
H. _____

6

lung
A. aortic arch
B. trachea
H. left main bronchus
J. pulmonary vessels
K. normal lung

Note that on CT, as on the x-ray, the tapering peripheral vessels are beyond the resolution of the CT scan.

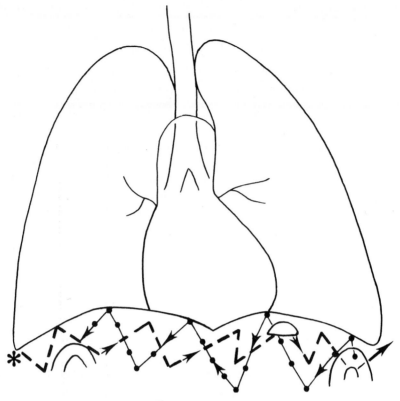

Figure 3–5A

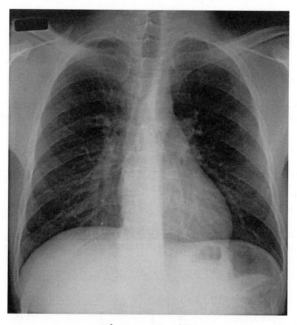

Figure 3–5B

In order to maximize your accuracy, you must have an organized search pattern. Start reading every radiograph—chest or otherwise—by scanning the areas of least interest *first,* working toward the more important areas. You are less likely to miss secondary but important findings this way. For the chest x-ray, start in the upper abdomen, then look at the thoracic cage (soft tissues and bones), then the mediastinal structures, and, lastly, the lung. Look at each lung individually and then compare left lung and right lung.

7

Arrange the following in viewing sequence:

A. mediastinum _____ D. lungs—bilateral _____

B. lung—unilateral _____ E. thorax _____

C. abdomen _____

My way
1. Alignment   4. Lungs
2. Exposure   5. Mediastinum
3. Order   6. Thorax
*   7. Abdomen*

AE man are there many lung lesions?

7

Correct sequence:

1 = Abdomen

2 = Thorax (soft tissues and bones)

3 = Mediastinum

4 = Lung—unilateral

5 = Lungs—bilateral

Are There Many Lung Lesions?

Abdomen. In Figure 3–5A, start in the right upper quadrant (*) and scan across the upper abdomen several times. Normal gas-containing structures are the stomach and the hepatic and splenic flexures of the colon. The liver is always visible and the spleen is often visible.

8

Scan the abdomen in Figure 3–5B.

A. The gas collection just below the heart = _____ .

B. The gas collection lateral to A = _____ .

C. The homogeneous density below the right diaphragm

= _____ .

D. The _____ diaphragm is higher. This is normal.

8

A. stomach bubble

B. splenic flexure of colon

C. liver

D. right

Clinical Pearl: Upper abdominal disease (subphrenic abscess, perforated viscus, pancreatitis, cholecystitis) may mimic lung disease clinically. Similarly, basilar lung disease (pneumonia, pleurisy) may mimic upper abdominal disease.

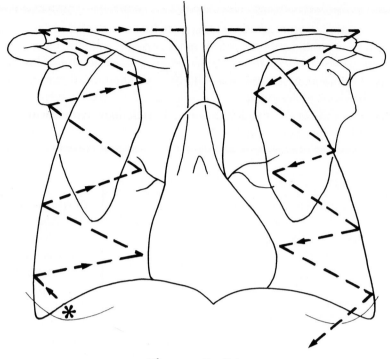

Figure 3–6A

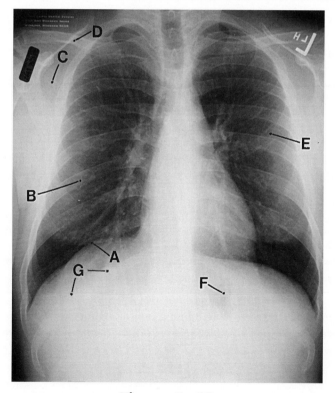

Figure 3–6B

Thorax. In Figure 3–6A, start at the right base (*), looking at the soft tissues (muscles, breast, etc.) of the chest wall, the ribs, and the shoulder girdle in sequence. Finish by reversing the order down the left side. These structures are represented in Figure 3–6B. Note that the posterior ribs descend from medial to lateral, while the anterior ribs descend from lateral to medial.

9

In Figure 3–6B, identify the following structures:

A. _____

B. _____

C. _____

D. _____

E. _____

F. _____

G. _____

9

A. *right breast*

B. *posterior ribs*

C. *scapula*

D. *clavicle*

E. *anterior ribs*

F. *stomach*

G. *liver*

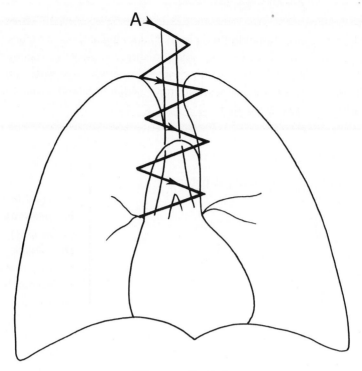

Figure 3–7A

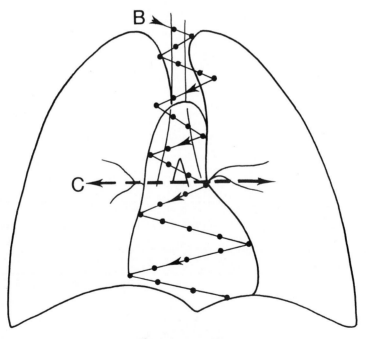

Figure 3–7B

Mediastinum. An organized search of the mediastinum is complicated because there are multiple overlapping structures. Start with a global look at the mediastinum for contour abnormalities (e.g., focal or diffuse widening), then follow with a directed search. Figure 3–7A and B show three searches of the mediastinum. A = trachea and carina; B = aorta and heart; C = hilum.

10

Return to Figure 3–2A and identify the following structures in the order of your mediastinal search:

I _____

II _____

III _____

IV _____

V _____

VI _____

VII _____

10

I. *trachea*

II. *carina*

III. *aortic knob (arch)*

IV. *ascending aorta*

V. *descending aorta*

VI. *heart*

VII. *hilum*

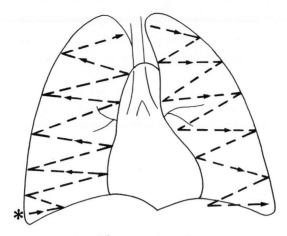

Figure 3–8A

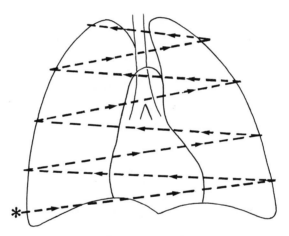

Figure 3–8B

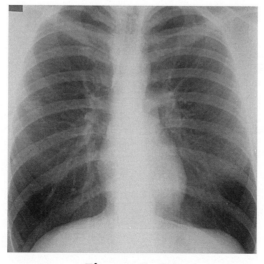

Figure 3–9A

Lungs. Most chest x-rays are ordered to evaluate lung disease, so the lungs are examined last. They are so important that we search the lungs twice. Start in the right costophrenic angle (*) as outlined in Figure 3–8A, examining the right and then left lung and costophrenic angle. The second look involves a side-by-side comparison of the lungs (Fig. 3–8B). This should also give you a second look at costophrenic angles and the hilum. Practice this search pattern in Figure 3–9A. **Are There Many Lung Lesions?**

11

See anything abnormal in Figure 3–9A? The abnormality is subtle. Compare side to side. The change should be obvious (it is to me anyway). There is a nodule in the _____ .

11

right midlung laterally, over fourth anterior rib (Who said this would be easy?)

Clinical Pearl: The old x-ray is your best friend. Radiologists always look at old films when available. You should too. They help you detect new disease and evaluate for change in preexisting disease. In Figure 3–9B, one year earlier, the nodule is barely visible *(arrow)*.

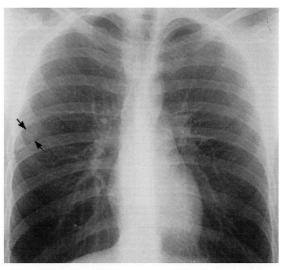

Figure 3–9B

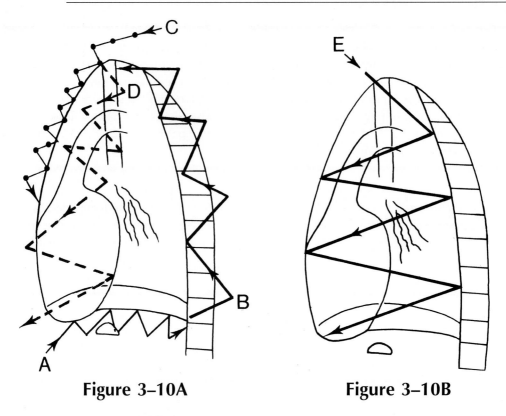

Figure 3–10A   **Figure 3–10B**

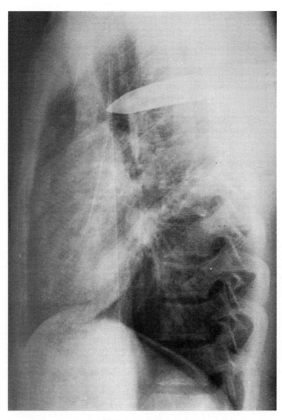

Figure 3–11

12

For the novice, subtle, and not so subtle, abnormalities are easy to miss. In searching the lungs, three helpful strategies to minimize oversights are 1) searching the lungs individually, 2) searching the lungs _____ , and 3) taking advantage of _____ , if available.

12

side by side
old radiographs

The lateral is a valuable but often ignored radiograph. Don't ignore it! The search pattern is identical (ATMLL). In Figure 3–10A, start by searching below the diaphragm (A). Continue at the lower spine (B), searching the soft tissues and bones posteriorly, then anteriorly (C). Return to the trachea and work your way down the mediastinum (D). In Figure 3–10B, crisscross the superimposed lungs and costophrenic angles.

13

Repeat the search in Figure 3–11. This patient is complaining of [dyspnea/cough/back pain] because of _____ .

13
back pain
knife in back

How to tell who used the x-ray folder last? *A radiologist:* the PA and lateral films are in chronological order. *An internist:* the PA's are in chronological order in the front and the laterals are in random order in the back. *A surgeon:* all films are in random order. *An orthopedist:* half the films are missing.

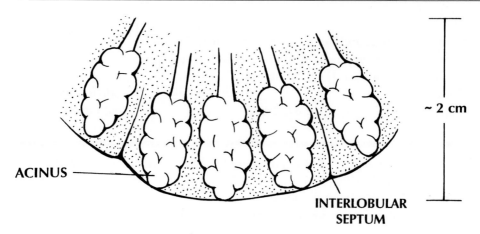

ACINUS

INTERLOBULAR
SEPTUM

~ 2 cm

Figure 3–12

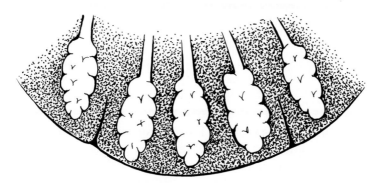

Figure 3–13A

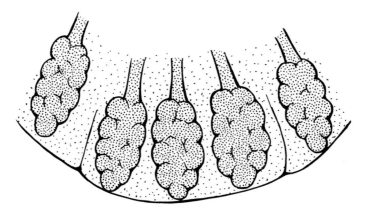

Figure 3–13B

14

A bit of terminology before we proceed. You have probably heard the terms "alveolar" and "interstitial lung disease." This is the area that causes the most confusion among nonradiologists and dyspepsia among semantic purists. In the simplest terms, the lung consists of air sacs and supporting structures. These air sacs are called _____ , contain air, and are _____ on the x-ray. Figure 3–12 shows alveoli arranged into acini around terminal airways. Several acini form a secondary pulmonary lobule, the basic unit of lung function and gross morphology.

An Acinus is the terminal respiratous unit (Robbins).

15

Supporting the alveoli are vessels, lymphatics, bronchi, and connective tissue. This support framework is known collectively as the _____ of the lung. On a normal chest x-ray, the branching pulmonary vessels (hilar vessels) are our only look at the interstitium. They branch and taper and become invisible in the outer third of the lung—not because they don't exist peripherally, but because they are _____ .

16

If a disease affects only the interstitium, the interstitial tissue around the small vessels or interlobular septa will [thicken/thin] and they will become [more visible/less visible] at the periphery of the lung. Since the air in the alveoli is hardly affected, the lung still appears well aerated.

14

alveoli
radiolucent (black) (invisible)

15

interstitium

too small to resolve ("tiny" for you non–science majors)

16

thicken
more visible

Figure 3–13A shows thickened interstitium and normal aeration. Compare with normal (Fig. 3–12).

17

If fluid or tissue (blood, edema, mucus, tumor, etc.) fills the air sacs, the lungs will become [radiodense/radiolucent]. The interstitial markings will be [more/less] visible within the alveolar consolidation. Figure 3–13B demonstrates alveolar or airspace consolidation, while Figure 3–13A demonstrates _____ .

17

radiodense
less

interstitial thickening

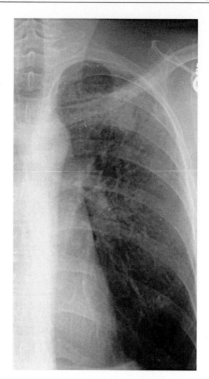

Figure 3–14A

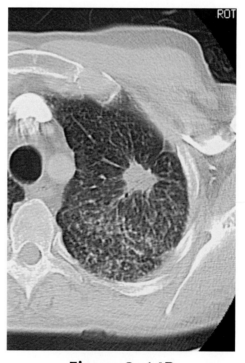

Figure 3–14B

Figure 3–14A shows normal lung at the base, prominent interstitium in the upper half, and a focal alveolar density just below the clavicle. Figure 3–14B, a CT through lung apex, shows interstitial thickening and an area of airspace consolidation. Compare with a normal CT (Fig. 3–4A).

That's it, alveolar and interstitial disease—grossly oversimplified—but a good place to start. Try to analyze each abnormal x-ray with these patterns in mind.

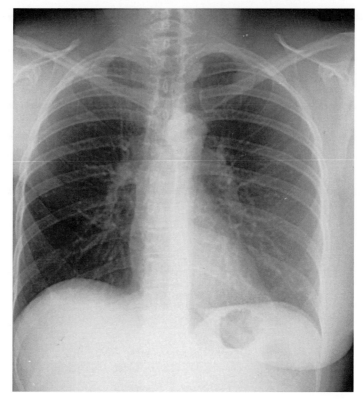

Figure 3–15

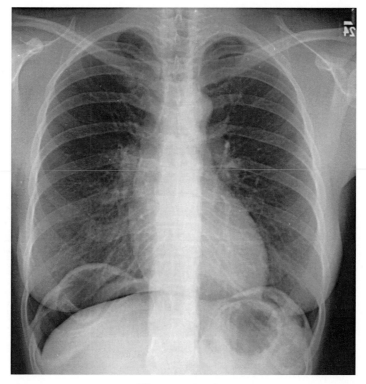

Figure 3–16

REVIEW

I

Chest x-ray reading sequence:

A =
T =
M =
L =
L =   *AR MAN*

(Are There Many Lung Lesions?)

II

With the interstitial pattern, the lungs appear well _____ , but the lung markings are _____ . Conversely, with the alveolar pattern the individual lung markings are _____ , because the surrounding lung is _____ .

III

Search Figure 3–15 systematically. Then answer the questions below:

A. Which lung is more radiolucent? _____

B. What is the cause of the density difference? _____

IV

Search Figure 3–16 systematically. Then answer the questions below:

A. The lungs are _____ .

B. The patient's pain is due to _____ .

I

Abdomen
Thorax
Mediastinum
Lung—unilateral
Lungs—bilateral

II

aerated
thick
invisible
airless (consoli-dated) (radiodense)

III

A. right
B. right mastectomy; there is less x-ray absorption, more film blackening

IV

A. normal
B. perforated stomach or bowel (free air under diaphragms)

(If you got these answers, great, you searched systematically. If not, review #7–12.)

Lobar Anatomy

A fingertip knowledge of lobar and segmental anatomy is indispensable for understanding patterns of lung disease. Some diseases have lobar or segmental distributions; others do not. Some are even limited to specific segments. Understanding the lobes and segments is also important for orientation at bronchoscopy, in planning surgery and radiation therapy, and in prescribing postural drainage for pneumonias and abscesses.

1

We challenge you to test your anatomic recall:

(a) Which lung is the smaller? _____

(b) Name the lobes of the right lung. _____ ,
_____ , and _____

(c) Name the lobes of the left lung. _____
and _____

1

(a) *left, because heart is on left*

(b) *upper, middle, lower*

(c) *upper, lower (lingula is part of LUL)*

2

The inner thoracic wall is lined by the _____ pleura, while each lobe is surrounded by the _____ pleura. The space between the visceral and parietal pleura is cleverly named the _____ .

2

parietal

visceral
pleural space

3

The space between the lobes, where the _____ pleural surfaces touch is called the interlobular fissure or septa. Since the visceral pleura is less than 1 mm thick, the x-ray beam must strike it parallel to its surface if it is to be visible on the radiograph. If a fissure is not _____ to the x-ray beam, it will not be visualized.

3

visceral

INTERLOBAR ?

parallel

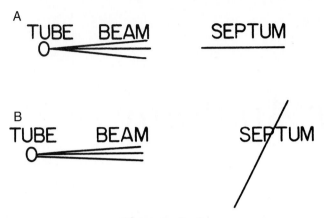

Figure 4–1

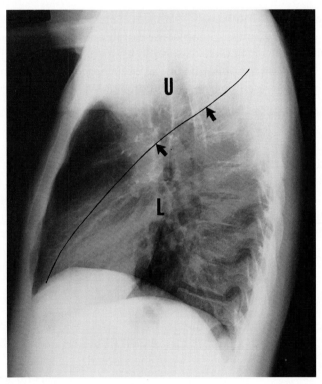

Figure 4–2

4

In Figure 4–1*A*, the x-ray beam is [perpendicular/parallel] to the septum (fissure). The fissure [will/will not] be visible on the radiograph.

In Figure 4–1*B*, the x-ray beam is [oblique/parallel] to the visceral pleural surfaces. The fissure [will/will not] be visible on the radiograph.

5

Figure 4–2 shows that in the left lung, the upper lobe (U) is separated from the lower lobe (L) by the _____ (*arrows*). The major fissure is [perpendicular/parallel] to the x-ray beam only in the lateral projection. (For your benefit, the fissures are often outlined in black or illustrated because they are difficult to reproduce.)

6

The _____ fissure runs obliquely downward from about the level of the fifth thoracic vertebra posteriorly to the _____ inferiorly, at a point just short of the anterior chest wall.

7

The oblique (major, vertical) fissure is not visible on the normal frontal projection because *(choose one)*:
(a) It is often anatomically absent.
(b) It is not parallel to the x-ray beam.
(c) It has the same roentgen density as lung tissue.

8

In the right lung, the major (oblique) fissure separates the upper and middle lobes from the _____ . On the left, it separates the _____ .

4
parallel
will

oblique
will not

5

major (oblique) (vertical)
fissure
parallel

6
major (oblique) (vertical)

diaphragm

7

(b) It is not parallel to the x-ray beam.

8

lower lobe
upper and lower lobes

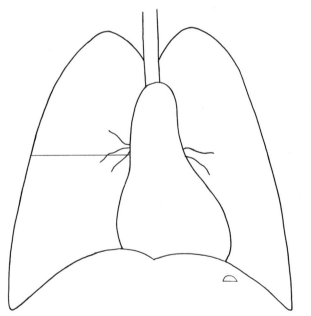

Figure 4–3A

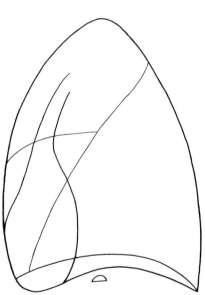

Figure 4–3B

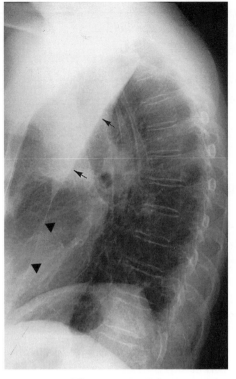

Figure 4–4A

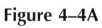

Figure 4–4B

The fissure normally appears as a thin white line (pleura surrounded by air) as in Figure 4–3A *(arrowheads)*. There are two exceptions. If a lobe is consolidated, the fissure appears as an edge. In Figure 4–3A, the lower fissure is a line *(arrowheads)*, but the upper fissure is an edge *(arrows)* because the upper lobe is airless. If pleural fluid enters a fissure, the fissure thickens. Note the thick major fissure and normal minor *(arrow)* fissure in Figure 4–3B.

9

The minor (horizontal) fissure separates the right middle lobe from the [right upper/right lower] lobe. In the erect patient, the minor fissure is usually horizontal. It is [parallel/perpendicular] to the floor (Fig. 4–3B and Fig. 4–4A and B). This fissure should be visible in the [frontal/lateral/both] view(s).

right upper
parallel

both

10

In many people, the minor fissure is not perfectly horizontal. The anterior portion or the entire fissure slopes downward, making it invisible in the _____ projection. In others, the minor fissure is anatomically incomplete and not visible in one or both views.

frontal

Just to confuse you a little, a small percentage of people have a left minor fissure between the lingula and the rest of the upper lobe. Watch for it.

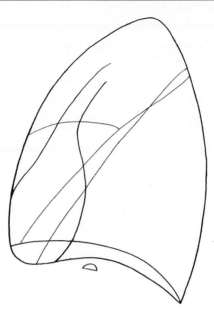

Figure 4–5

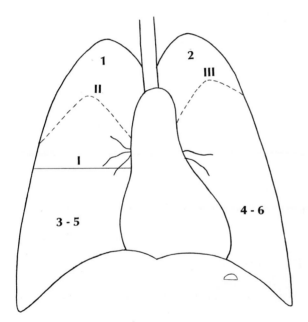

Figure 4–6A

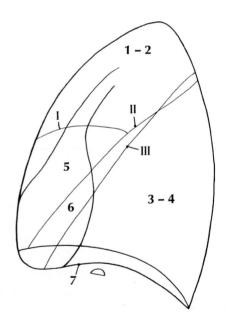

Figure 4–6B

11

On the lateral film (Fig. 4–5), the minor fissure starts at the _____ wall and ends on the _____ fissure. This helps us distinguish the right from the left major fissure on the lateral view.

11

anterior chest/right major

In the lateral view, it may still be difficult to tell the two major fissures apart. Here is a simple method: The left major fissure ends on the left diaphragm. The left diaphragm is usually lower, usually has the stomach bubble immediately beneath it, and is not visible anteriorly because the bottom of the heart rests on it (Fig. 4–5).

12

Identify the fissures in Figure 4–6A and B

(a) I   = _____

(b) II = _____

(c) III = _____

12

(a) minor fissure

(b) right major fissure

(c) left major fissure

13

Identify the following lobes in Figure 4–6A and B:

(a) 1 and 2 = _____

(b) 3 and 5 = _____

(c) 3 and 4 = _____

(d) 5 = _____

(e) 6 = _____

(f) 7 = _____

13

(a) upper lobes

(b) right lower and middle lobes

(c) lower lobes

(d) right middle lobe

(e) lingula

(f) left diaphragm

Note: On the frontal view (Fig. 4–6A), the superior portions of the lower lobes rise to the level of the aortic arch *(dashed lines)*.

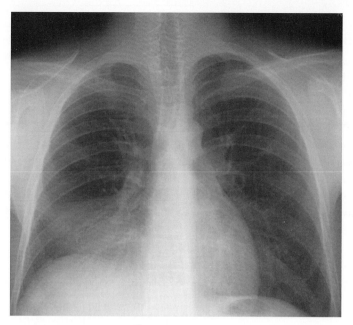

Figure 4–7A

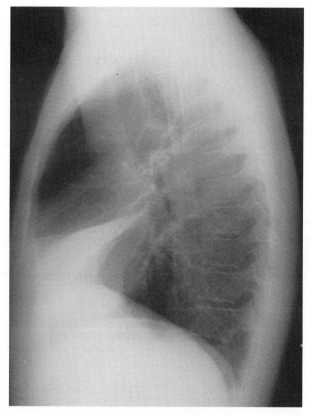

Figure 4–7B

14
In Figure 4–7*A* and *B*, there is [alveolar/interstitial] disease located in the _____ lobe.

14
alveolar
right middle

Clinical Pearl: Lobar pneumonia is usually bacterial in origin, due to *Streptococcus pneumoniae* or *Klebsiella*. *Mycoplasma* or *Legionella* infections occasionally cause lobar consolidation.

On radiographs, fissures are seen when parallel to the x-ray beam. On CT, structures are best seen when perpendicular to the scan plane. The major fissures *(arrows)* are usually visible on CT (Fig. 4–8). The minor fissure is in the scan plane and is not visible.

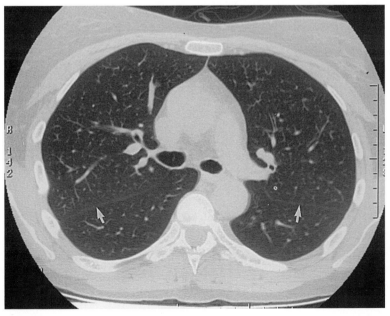

Figure 4–8

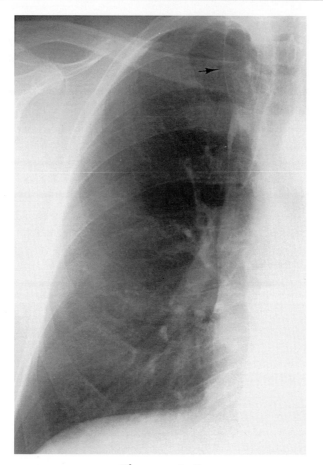

Figure 4–9

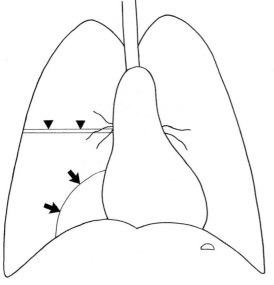

Figure 4–10A

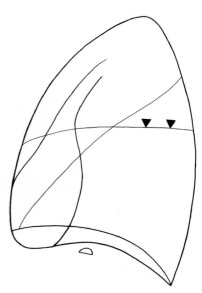

Figure 4–10B

15

What about other fissures? There are three accessory fissures seen in less than 5% of normal people. The azygos fissure (Fig. 4–9) is formed by an anomalous development of the azygos vein. The vein "migrates through" the medial right upper lobe, dragging visceral and parietal pleura with it. The azygos lobe is separated from the rest of the upper lobe by the azygos _____ *(arrow)*.

16

The azygos fissure separates a variable amount of the upper medial region of the _____ lobe. This portion of the lung is called the _____ lobe. This interesting information is of [great/little] clinical importance.

17

Figure 4–10*A* shows the position of another anomalous fissure *(arrows)*, the inferior accessory fissure. It separates the medial basal segment of the _____ lobe from the remainder of the lobe.

18

The azygos and inferior accessory fissures run in an anterior-posterior plane. They are visible in the [frontal/lateral/both] view(s).

19

The third accessory fissure is the superior accessory fissure. In Figure 4–10*A* and *B*, this fissure *(arrowheads)* is in the same plane and posterior to the _____ fissure. It should be visible in the [frontal/lateral/both] view(s). It often superimposes on the minor fissure in the _____ view.

20

The superior accessory fissure divides the _____ lobe into two portions: the basal segments and the [superior/inferior/apical] segment.

15

Azygos Fissure

fissure

16
right upper
azygos
little

17

Inferior Accessory Fissure

right lower

18

frontal

19

Superior Accessory Fissure

minor
both

frontal

20
right lower

superior

Train yourself to look for the fissures on *every* roentgenogram of the chest. They help to localize disease in the lung. As we shall see, displacement of the fissures is the most reliable sign of lobar collapse.

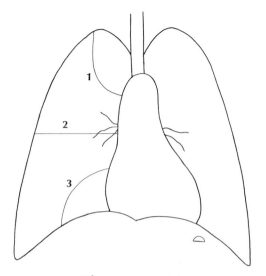

Figure 4–11A

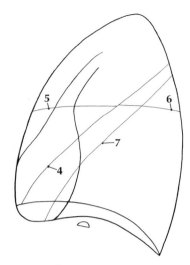

Figure 4–11B

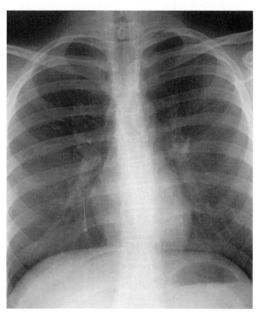

Figure 4–12A

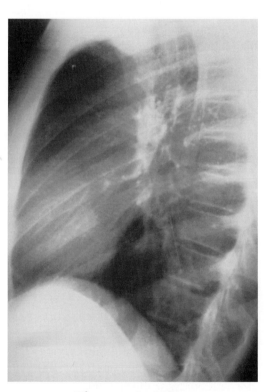

Figure 4–12B

REVIEW

I

Identify the fissures in Figure 4–11*A* and *B*:

(1) _____
(2) _____ or _____
(3) _____
(4) _____
(5) _____
(6) _____
(7) _____

I

(1) azygos
(2) minor (or) superior accessory
(3) inferior accessory
(4) right major
(5) minor
(6) superior accessory
(7) left major

II

The only fissures visible on the frontal and lateral view are the _____ fissure and the _____ accessory fissure. Why? _____

II

minor/superior
Parallel to beam, in both projections (both horizontal)

III

An unlucky seamstress gasped at the wrong moment. Carefully scan Figure 4–12*A* and *B*; then answer the following questions:
(a) What is the abnormality? _____
(b) In what lobe is it located? _____

III

(a) aspirated a pin
(b) right lower lobe

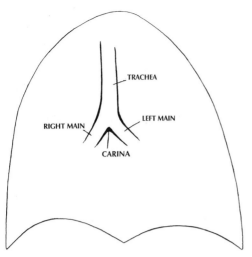

Figure 5–1

Figure 5–2

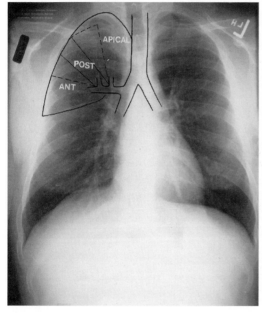

Figure 5–3A

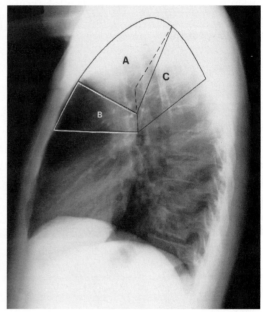

Figure 5–3B

Segmental Anatomy

5

Each lung is divided into lobes and each lobe is divided into segments. Each segment is supplied by its own bronchus, which is called a segmental bronchus. We will learn the anatomy of the tracheobronchial tree and the segments together. (One less chapter you have to read, one less chapter I have to write.)

1

Study Figure 5–1. You should be familiar with this anatomy already. The trachea bifurcates at the _____ , into the right and left _____ bronchi. The right then divides into [one/two/three] lobar bronchi, while the left divides into [one/two/three].

1

carina
main (or main stem)
three—upper, middle, lower
two—upper, lower (lingula part of upper lobe)

2

Let's start with the right upper lobe (RUL). In Figure 5–2, the RUL bronchus comes off at about the level of the carina. It divides into _____ segmental bronchi.

2

three

Over the years, several numbering systems have been used to describe the segmental bronchi. They are difficult to remember and seldom used. I prefer the anatomic names. They are logical and one less thing to memorize. Understanding lasts longer than memorization. Remember that!

In Figure 5–2, the diagram shows the three RUL segmental bronchi described by location: apical (#1); anterior (#2); posterior (#3). The numbers are the Boyden system, for those who prefer numbers to names.

3

Figure 5–3A illustrates the overlap of the three segments on the frontal radiograph. Use Figure 5–2 and Figure 5–3A to name the segments on the lateral x-ray (Fig. 5–3B).

A _____ B _____ C _____

3

A. apical
B. anterior
C. posterior

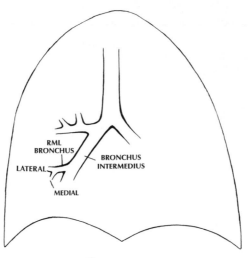

Figure 5–4

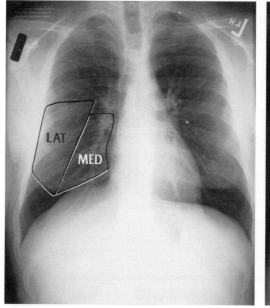

Figure 5–5A

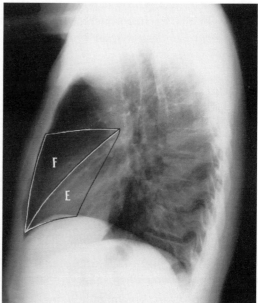

Figure 5–5B

Clinical Pearl: Reactivation (postprimary) tuberculosis is usually in the apical (#1) and/or posterior (#3) segments of the upper lobes. In the anterior segment (#2), postprimary TB is rare, whereas cancer is fairly common in older adults.

4

In Figure 5–4, the bronchus intermedius is a continuation of the right _____ bronchus after the takeoff of the _____ .

4

main
RUL bronchus

5

In Figure 5–4, the right middle lobe (RML) bronchus arises from the _____ . It courses anteriorly and divides into two segmental bronchi: the lateral segment (#4) and the _____ segmental (#5) bronchi.

5

bronchus intermedius

medial

6

Figure 5–5A shows the overlapping RML segments. Use Figure 5–4 and Figure 5–5A to name the segments in the lateral projection, Figure 5–5B.

E _____   F _____

6

E = medial
F = lateral

7

In Figure 5–5A and B, the _____ segment (#4) is bordered by the _____ fissure superiorly on both the PA and lateral. The _____ segment (#5) lies against the right heart border, medially, and against the _____ fissure, posteriorly.

7

lateral / minor

minor medial

medial/major

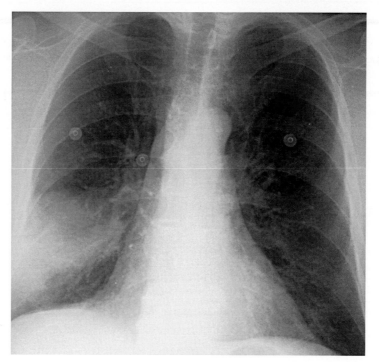

Figure 5–6

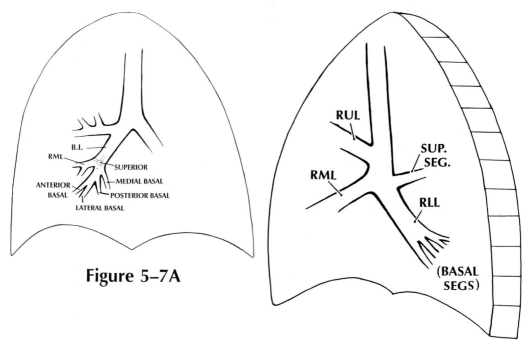

Figure 5–7A

Figure 5–7B

Figure 5–6 shows a segmental pneumonia in the lateral segment of the middle lobe. The sharp upper margin is the minor fissure. It does not make contact with the right heart border, which is easily seen.

8

Name all of the RUL and RML segments:

#1 _____

#2 _____

#3 _____

#4 _____

#5 _____

8

#1 apical—RUL

#2 anterior—RUL

#3 posterior—RUL

#4 lateral—RML

#5 medial—RML

9

The right lower lobe (RLL) bronchus is the direct continuation of the bronchus intermedius after the takeoff of the _____ bronchus (Fig. 5–7A and B).

9

RML

10

In Figure 5–7B, the lateral view shows the first segmental bronchus of the RLL arises posteriorly, just opposite the RML bronchus. It runs posteriorly to supply the superior segment (#6) of the right _____ lobe.

10

lower

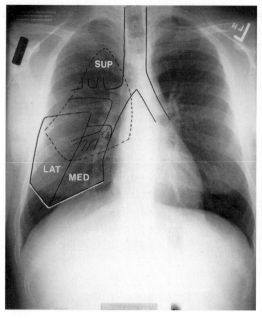

Figure 5–8A

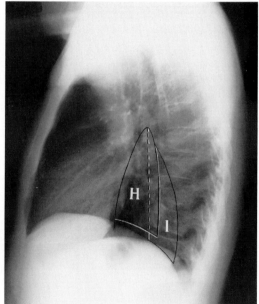

Figure 5–8B

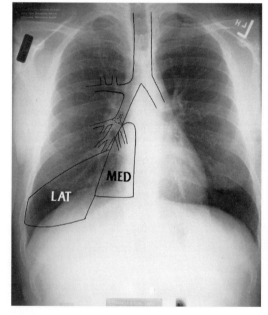

Figure 5–9A

Figure 5–9B

11

Figure 5–8A and B show the anatomic position of the superior segment of the RLL. On the frontal view (Fig. 5–8A), the superior segment of the RLL, overlaps the _____ and _____ lobes. On the lateral view, identify:

E _____

F _____

G _____

middle/upper

E. RML, medial
F. RML, lateral
G. RLL, superior segment

12

The four remaining segmental bronchi supply the four *basal* segments of the RLL. They are named for their location at the lung base (see Fig. 5–7). Two basal segments are located ventrally (anteriorly), the medial (#7) and the anterior (#8). Two basal segments are located dorsally (posteriorly), the _____ (#9) and _____ (#10).

lateral/posterior

13

The two basal segments that contact the major fissure are the _____ and the _____ . The two that contact the posterior thoracic wall are the _____ and the _____ .

medial/anterior
posterior/lateral

14

Figure 5–9A and B show the position of the medial basal (#7) and the lateral basal (#9). In the lateral view, identify

H _____ and I _____ .

H. medial basal
I. lateral basal

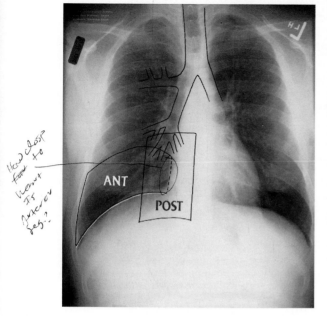

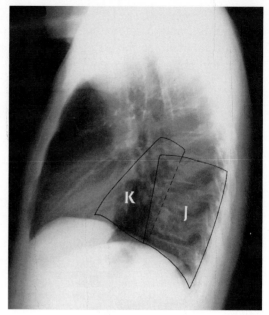

Figure 5–10A

Figure 5–10B

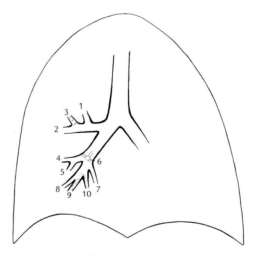

Figure 5–11

15

Figure 5–10*A* and 5–10*B* show the remaining basal segments: _____ (#8) and _____ (#10). In the lateral, identify J _____ and K _____ .

15

#8 anterior basal
#10 posterior basal
J. posterior basal
K. anterior basal

16

In Figure 5–9*B* and Figure 5–10*B*, which basal segments border on the major fissure? _____ Which border on the minor fissure? _____

16

medial, anterior
none

17

Return to Figure 4–11*A* and *B*. The pin is in the _____ segment of the RLL.

17

posterior basal (#10)

Clinical Pearl: The posterior segment (#3) of the upper lobes and the superior segments (#6) and posterior basal segments (#10) of the lower lobes are the most gravity-dependent segments. Aspiration pneumonitis, foreign body aspiration, and abscess often occur in these segments.

18

Name all the segmental bronchi of the right lung indicated in Figure 5–11.

#1 _____
#2 _____
#3 _____
#4 _____
#5 _____
#6 _____
#7 _____
#8 _____
#9 _____
#10 _____

18

#1 apical RUL
#2 anterior RUL
#3 posterior RUL
#4 lateral RML
#5 medial RML
#6 superior RLL
#7 medial basal RLL
#8 anterior basal RLL
#9 lateral basal RLL
#10 posterior basal RLL

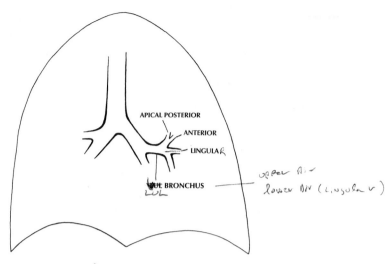

Figure 5–12

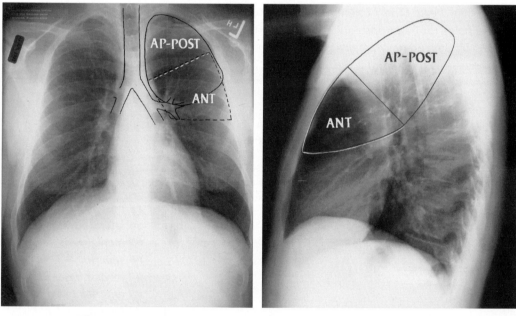

Figure 5–13A   **Figure 5–13B**

Basically, if you know the right lung segments, the left is easy. The differences between the two lungs are minor, so don't get discouraged. (There are basically two types of people, optimists and pessimists. The optimists are usually happy and the pessimists are usually right.)

19
First of all, there are only two lobes on the left, the _____ lobe and the _____ lobe. The homologue of the _____ is called the *lingula.* (Now whose bright idea was that?)

19

upper/lower

RML

20
Figure 5–12 shows that the first lobar bronchus arising from the left main bronchus is the left _____ bronchus. It branches into an upper division and lower division, which is called the _____

20

upper lobe

lingula

21
Figure 5–12 shows that the upper division bronchus divides only twice—into the combined apical posterior segment (#1 and #3) and the _____ segment (#2). The LUL apical-posterior segment is the equivalent of the apical and posterior segments of the RUL.

21

anterior

Figure 5–13*A* and *B* shows that in the upper division, the LUL segments are very similar to the RUL segments (Fig. 5–3).

22
The RML bronchus arises from the _____ . There is no similar bronchus on the left. The lingula is the continuation of the _____ bronchus just distal to the upper division bronchus.

22
bronchus intermedius

LUL

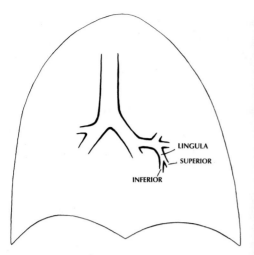

Figure 5–14

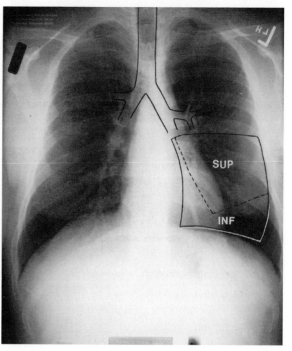

Figure 5–15A

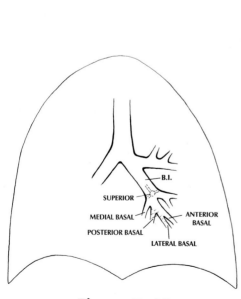

Figure 5–16

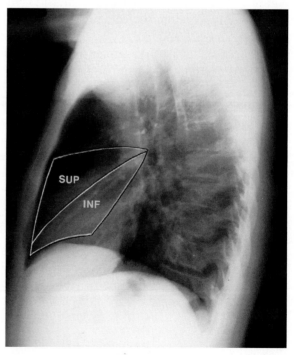

Figure 5–15B

23

Figure 5–14 shows that the lower or _____ division of the LUL is subdivided into two segments: the superior (#4) and the _____ (#5). These are similar in location to the lateral and medial segments of the RML. One more quirk of anatomic nomenclature to have to deal with!

23

lingula

inferior

The lingula segments are shown in Figure 5–15. The inferior segment (#5) of the lingula and the medial segment (#5) of the RML contact the heart medially and the major fissure posteriorly. The superior segment would contact the left minor fissure, if one existed.

24

Guess what? The LLL and the RLL segmental anatomies are similar. (Some authorities fuse the anterior [#8] and medial [#7] segments into one. Let's not; let's keep it simple.) Using what you have learned about the RLL, name the segments of the LLL illustrated in Figure 5–16:

#6 _____   #9 _____

#7 _____   #10 _____

#8 _____

24

#6 superior
#7 medial basal
#8 anterior basal
#9 lateral basal
#10 posterior basal

Clinical Pearl: In bedridden patients, secretions often accumulate in the posterior basal segments, causing atelectasis.

The bronchial and segmental anatomy, as presented, is "idealized." There are numerous minor variations in the origin of the bronchi and the size of the segments. The basic patterns, however, are generally recognizable.

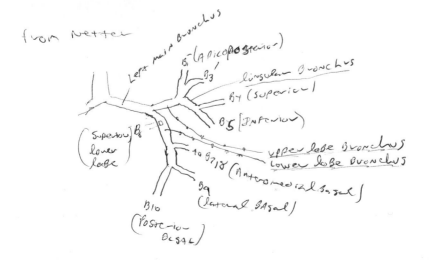

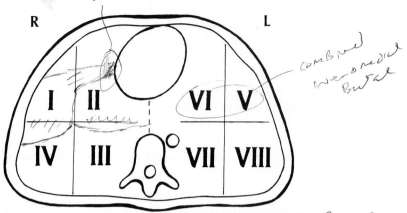

Figure 5–17 *See mine below ?*
or after 189

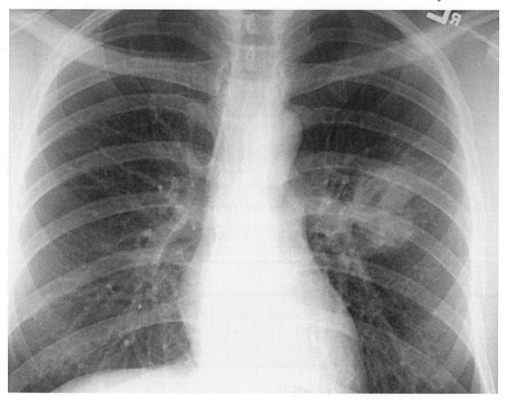

Figure 5–18A

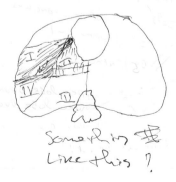

REVIEW

I

Figure 5–17 is an axial section through the basal segments. Identify the following segments:

I, V   _____

II, VI   _____

III, VII   _____

IV, VIII   _____

II

Using recall or the figures in this chapter, name the described segment(s):

A located just below minor fissure: _____

B located just above minor fissure: _____

C located adjacent to heart: _____ and _____

D contact diaphragm: _____

III

In Figure 5–18, the patient has pneumonia in the _____ segment of the _____ lobe.

I

I, V anterior basal

II, VI medial basal

III, VII posterior basal

IV, VIII lateral basal

II

A. *RML—lateral segment*

B. *RUL—anterior segment*

C. *RML—medial segment/ lingula—inferior segment*

D. *all basal segments*

III

superior/LLL

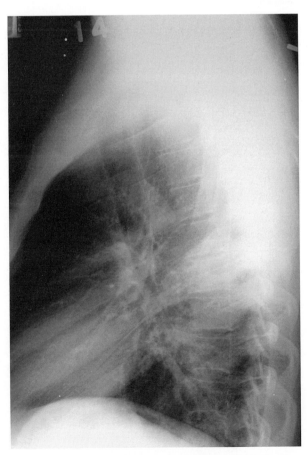

Figure 5–18B

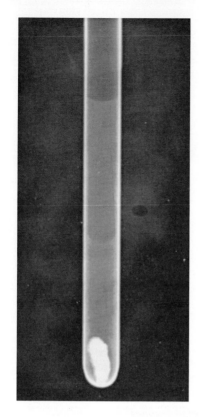

Figure 6–1

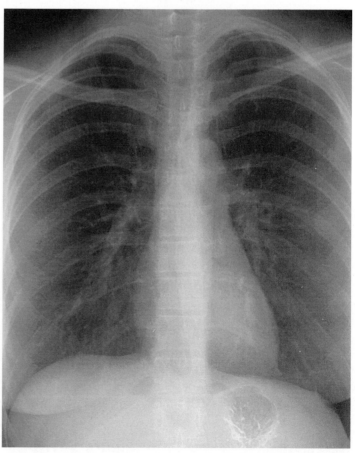

Figure 6–2

The Silhouette Sign

If part of the lung is radiodense (alveolar pattern, consolidated, water density, airless), it can affect our ability to see adjacent structures. We can use these changes to help us detect and localize disease in the lung. This chapter will discuss how disease in different lobes and segments affects the appearance of adjacent organs.

1

There are four basic radiographic densities. In order of increasing radiodensity, they are: gas, _____ , _____ and _____ .

1

fat, soft tissue (water), metal (bone)

Figure 6–1 shows a test tube containing, from top down, air, oil (fat), water, and metal. Calcium is the prime example of metal density *normally* found in the body. Note the sharp interface between densities.

2

Anatomic structures are recognized on the x-ray by their density differences. These four basic densities keep the radiologist in business. A normal chest film, Figure 6–2, shows them as the _____ density of the heart, muscles, and blood; the _____ density of the ribs; the _____ density of the lungs; and the fat density, which may be seen around the muscles (not shown).

2

water (soft tissue)
metal (bone)
gas (air)

In Figure 6–2, the heart, aorta, and diaphragms have sharp margins because they are all water density in direct contact with air density lung. Barium (metal density) and air in the stomach accentuate the gastric mucosa, which is soft tissue density.

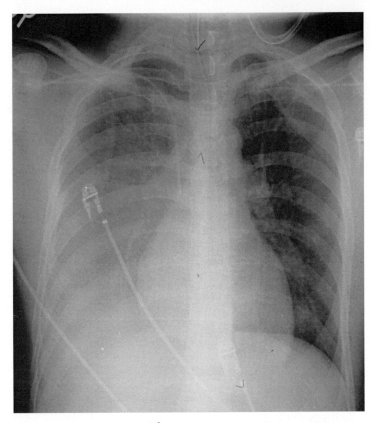

Figure 6–3

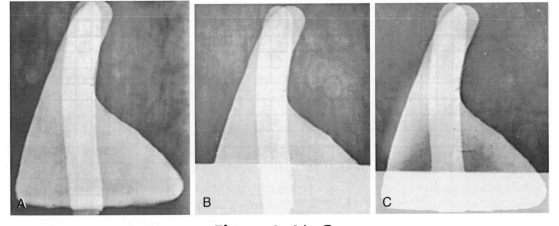

Figure 6–4A–C

3

The trachea, which is _____ density, can be differentiated from the mediastinum, which is _____ density. The liver and diaphragm cannot be separated because both are _____ density and in _____ .

3
air
soft tissue (water)
soft tissue
direct contact

The heart, aorta, and blood— as well as the liver, spleen, and muscles—are all soft tissue density. So is diseased *airless* lung. Two substances of the same density, *in direct contact,* cannot be differentiated from each other on an x-ray. This phenomenon, the loss of the normal radiographic silhouette (contour), is called the *silhouette sign*.

In Figure 6–3, the right lower lobe is consolidated (airless) and the adjacent right diaphragm is not visible, the silhouette sign. The right heart border, still in contact with aerated right middle lobe, is visible.

4

Let's reinforce this concept. Figure 6–4 shows three x-rays of a model of the heart and aorta. In Figure 6–4*A*, the heart and ascending aorta are in one box and the aortic knob and descending aorta are in a second box, *behind the first.* In Figure 6–4*B*, some water has been poured into the anterior box. The lower heart borders have disappeared. The descending aorta is _____ . In Figure 6–4*C*, the water has been removed and placed in the posterior box. The lower heart border is _____ , while the lower aortic border is _____ . Why? _____

4
visible
visible
not visible
heart contacts air, low
aorta contacts water

5

An interface is not visible when two areas of [similar/ different] radiodensity touch. This is the _____ sign.

5
similar
silhouette

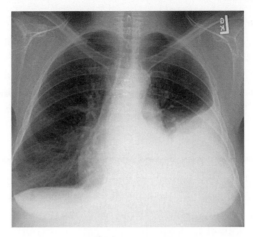

Figure 6–5

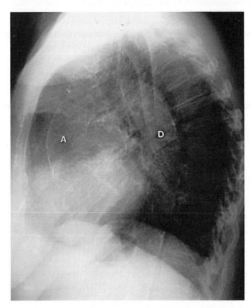

Figure 6–6A

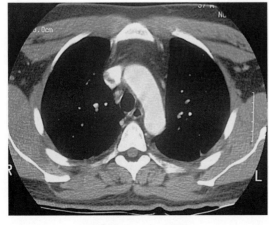

Figure 6–6B

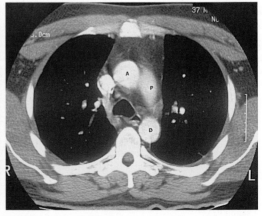

Figure 6–6C

Figure 6–5 demonstrates a large pleural effusion causing a silhouette sign of the diaphragm, the left heart border, and the descending aorta, similar to the model in Figure 6–4.

6

Now that you know what the silhouette sign is, what are you going to do with it? The silhouette sign helps diagnose and localize lung disease. If you know the position of intrathoracic structures, you can precisely localize the lung disease. The heart and ascending aorta are [anterior/posterior] structures. Conversely, the descending aorta is a(n) [anterior/posterior] structure. The aortic arch crosses the middle mediastinum from _____ on the right to _____ on the left.

6

anterior

posterior
anterior
posterior

Figure 6–6A is a lateral view of the chest with an atherosclerotic (calcified) aorta. The heart and ascending aorta (A) are anterior and the descending aorta (D) is posterior. Figure 6–6B is a CT scan taken through the aortic arch as it passes from right anterior to left posterior. In Figure 6–6C, the ascending aorta (A) is anterior and the descending aorta (D) is posterior. (P = pulmonary artery.)

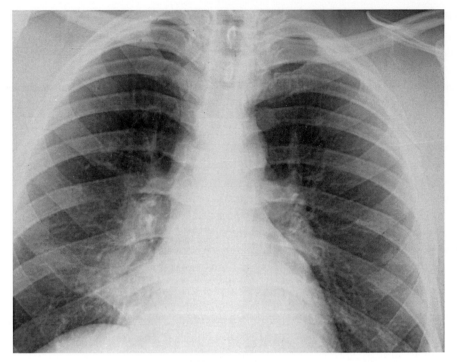

Figure 6–7

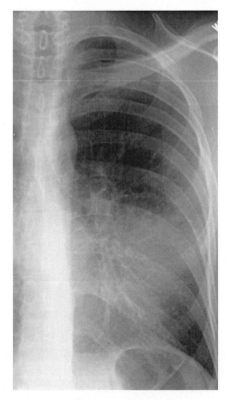

Figure 6–8A

7

Let's wrap this up. State the anterior or posterior location of each of the following:
(a) right heart border _____ (d) ascending aorta _____
(b) descending aorta _____ (e) aortic knob (arch) _____
(c) left heart border _____

7
(a) anterior
(b) posterior
(c) anterior
(d) anterior
(e) midposterior

8

Each lobe produces a characteristic silhouette sign we can take advantage of. The RML and lingula lie in anatomic contact with the _____ and _____ heart borders, respectively. All are [anterior/posterior]. In Figure 6–7, the left heart border is _____ and the right heart border is _____ . There must be consolidation (water density) in the _____ lobe.

8

right/left
anterior
visible
invisible (silhouette sign)
right middle

In Figure 6–8A, there is a silhouette sign of the left heart border. In Figure 6–8B, the CT shows the consolidated lingula adjacent to the left heart.

9

In Figure 6–7 and 6–8A, the diaphragms are [visible/invisible]. Why? _____

9
visible
diaphragms are adjacent to aerated lower lobes

10

Let's look at the lower lobes. They sit inferior and [anterior/posterior]. They are not in anatomic contact with the heart borders, which are anterior structures. Instead, they sit on the _____ , which are inferior structures.

10

posterior

diaphragms

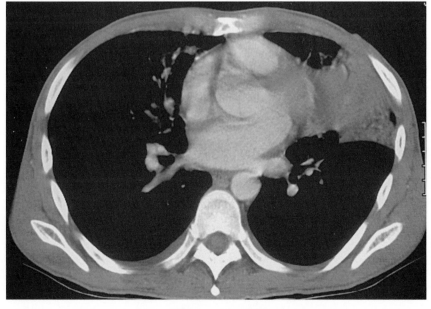

Figure 6–8B

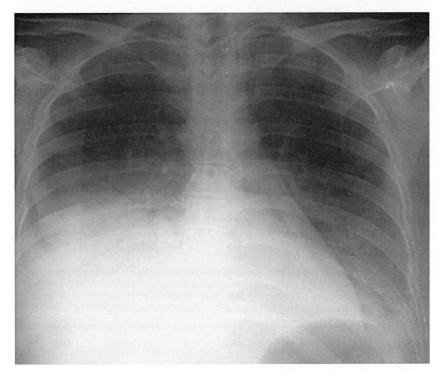

Figure 6–9

11

If only the right diaphragm is obscured, the disease is in the _____ . If the right heart border *and* the diaphragm are obscured, then there is consolidation of _____ and _____ .

11

RLL

RML/RLL

Figure 6–9 shows bilateral disease. On the right, there is a silhouette sign of the right heart and the diaphragm, indicating right middle and lower lobe disease. The left diaphragm and descending aorta are not visible due to a left lower lobe consolidation. The left heart border is sharp.

12

Airspace disease in either lower lobe will overlap the hilum and the heart border but will not obscure their silhouette because they are _____ .

12

not in direct contact

13

The descending aorta is not visible when there is _____ consolidation, as in Figure 6–9. Compare with Figure 6–12.

13

LLL

Clinical Pearl: In the ICU, left lower lobe atelectasis or pneumonia is frequent. Check the diaphragm and descending aorta through the heart on every film for a silhouette sign.

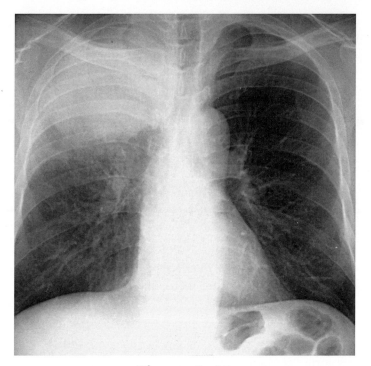

Figure 6–10

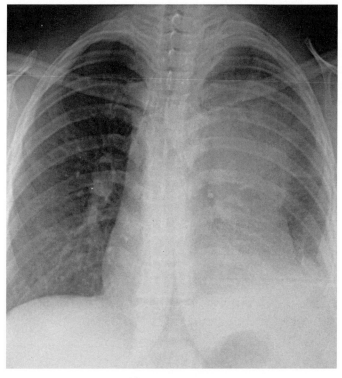

Figure 6–11

14

The upper right heart border and _____ aorta are anterior structures on the right. The descending aorta is _____ on the left. The trachea and the aortic knob are located in the _____ thorax.

14

ascending

posterior
mid — Mid thorax
trachea
Aortic knob

15

The RUL occupies the anterior and midthorax above the _____ fissure. RUL consolidation will cause a silhoutte sign of the _____ heart border and the right tracheal lung interface. Figure 6–10 shows RUL consolidation obscuring the mediastinum, aorta, and upper heart.

15

minor
upper right

16

LUL consolidation (upper division) will obliterate the _____ atrium, the aortic knob, and the _____ and _____ mediastinum. It may also obscure the proximal descending aorta. Figure 6–11 demonstrates the silhouette sign in LUL consolidation.

16

left
anterior/middle

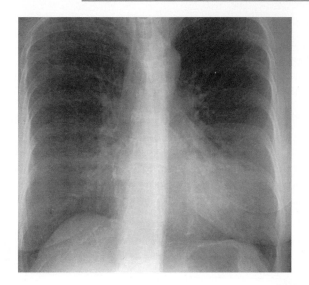

Figure 6–12

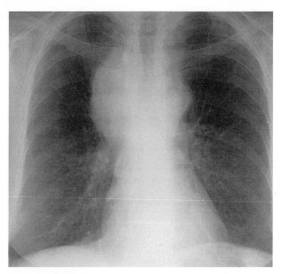

Figure 6–13

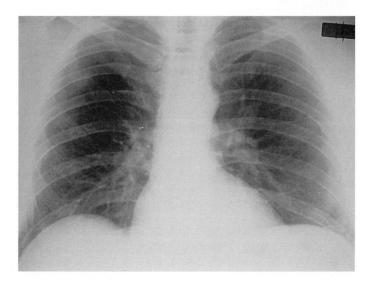

Figure 6–14

17

You have seen that a silhouette sign helps localize disease. Sometimes it actually helps detect disease. Study Figure 6–12 carefully. There are two subtle silhouette signs indicating disease in the _____ and _____ .

17

RML/lingula

A positive silhouette sign is very helpful. A negative silhouette sign does not assure that a given lobe is free of disease. Be careful!

You've learned that the silhouette sign applies to radiodense lung lesions. It also applies to soft tissue density mediastinal and pleural lesions. It applies whenever two structures of the *same* density are in contact.

18

If the lower descending thoracic aorta is not visible, the lesion causing this could lie in the _____ lobe, in the _____ pleural cavity, or in the adjacent (anterior/middle/posterior) mediastinum.

18

left lower
posterior
posterior

Review Figure 6–4 to see how an anterior pleural effusion affects the heart border and a posterior pleural effusion affects the descending aorta.

19

Figure 6–13 (p. 92) shows a mediastinal mass obscuring the ascending aorta and the trachea–lung interface. This large mass must be in the _____ and _____ mediastinum. What does it do to the trachea? _____ .

19

anterior/middle

compresses or narrows

Now that everything is clear—here come the exceptions. The silhouette sign may be misleading on an underpenetrated radiograph (a film that is too light). Figure 6–14 is an underpenetrated film. The left diaphragm and descending aorta are not visible through the heart. If you can't see the spine through the heart, the film is underpenetrated and a silhouette sign may be misleading.

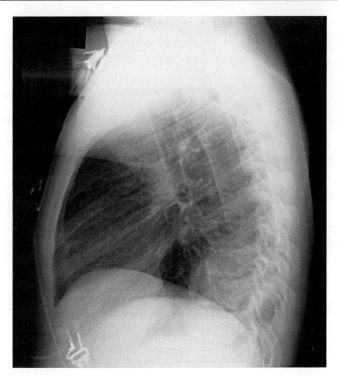

Figure 6–15

20

Another exception: Sometimes the right heart border over-lies the spine and doesn't protrude into the right lung. The _____ density of the spine hides the lung/heart interface.

20

bone (metal)

21

There is even a *normal* silhouette sign on the lateral radio-graph that we can use to advantage. The heart sits predom-inantly on the anterior [left/right] diaphragm. Both struc-tures are _____ density; therefore the [anterior/posterior] part of the left diaphragm is usually not visible. On the lateral, the right diaphragm is visible through the heart because _____ . This helps distinguish the left from the right diaphragm on the lateral.

21

left
soft tissue (water)
anterior

it contacts aerated lung

Figure 6–15 demonstrates two silhouette signs of the left diaphragm. The anterior one is due to the heart and the posterior one is due to pneumonia in the posterior basal segment of the LLL. Only the middle third of the left diaphragm is visible.

22

To obliterate the cardiovascular border or diaphragm, le-sions must be of _____ density. Calcified lesions and air-filled cavities next to these structures will not give a silhouette sign because _____ .

22

water (soft tissue)
they are of different roent-gen density (not water den-sity)

The silhouette sign is nearly always an abnormal finding. It is usually due to lung disease. It may be present even when you can't see the disease causing it. On every chest film you see from now on, look for the silhouette sign.

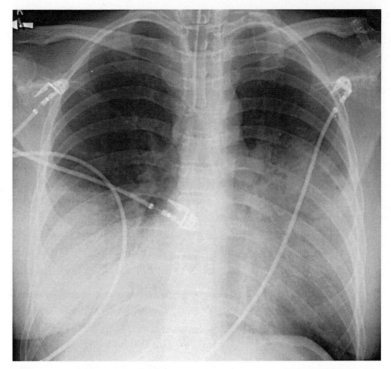

Figure 6–16

REVIEW

I

From the following descriptions of PA films, localize the lesion. Specify the segment, when possible.

(a) Lung consolidation obscures the left heart border: _____

(b) Lung consolidation obliterates the aortic knob: _____

(c) A right lung base pneumonia fails to obliterate the heart: _____

(d) A right lung base pneumonia obliterates the heart: _____

(e) An infiltrate obscures the descending aorta: _____

II

Let's review exceptions or false (+) silhouette signs.

A. A pseudosilhouette sign of the diaphragm may occur on an [over/under] penetrated radiograph. The radiograph is too [light/dark].

B. If the heart is positioned slightly to the left, the right heart border may not be seen because _____ .

C. On the lateral radiograph, the heart normally obscures the _____ .

III

In Figure 6–16, the patient has pneumococcal pneumonia. Without a lateral, determine which lobe(s) is (are) consolidated. _____

How did you decide? _____
_____ .

I

(a) lingula, inferior segment

(b) LUL, apical posterior segment

(c) RLL (probably)

(d) RML, medial segment

(e) LLL

II

A. under
light

B. it overlaps the spine

C. anterior left diaphragm

III

RML, RLL, lingula
right and left heart silhouette signs and right diaphragm silhouette sign

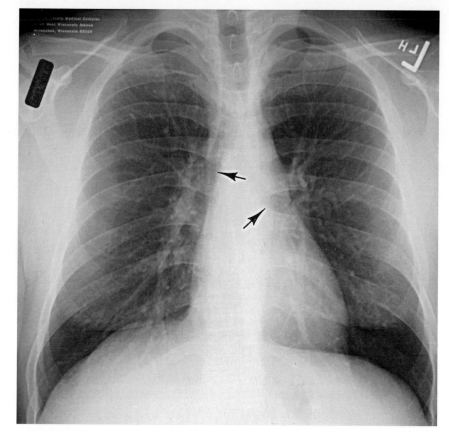

Figure 7–1

The Air Bronchogram Sign

On the normal chest x-ray, we see air in the trachea and proximal bronchi because they are surrounded by the soft tissue (water density) of the mediastinum. In the lungs, however, the bronchi are not visible. The only branching structures visible in the lungs are the pulmonary vessels (water density) surrounded by air.

1

The linear markings seen in the lungs are basically blood vessels, which are _____ density. Because bronchi have thin walls, contain air, and are surrounded by filled alveoli, the intraparenchymal bronchi [are/are not] visible on the normal chest x-ray.

1

water (soft tissue)

are not

In Figure 7–1, the branching pulmonary vessels are visible in the lung. The trachea and proximal main bronchi *(arrows)* are surrounded by mediastinal soft tissue and are visible. The peripheral bronchi are not visible.

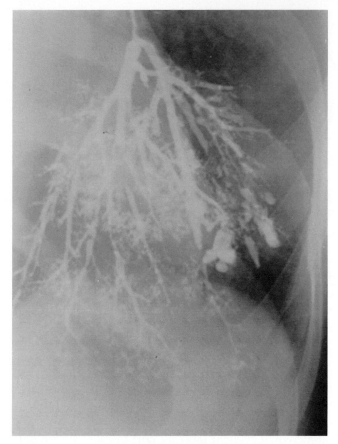

Figure 7–2A

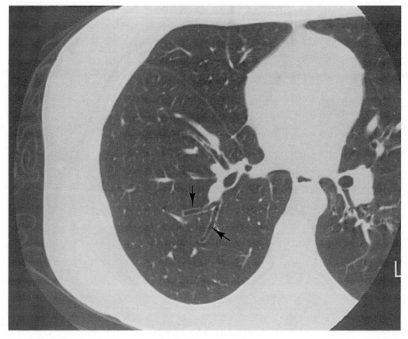

Figure 7–2B

2

In order to visualize the bronchi, we can instill an opaque material (iodinated oil) into the bronchial lumen. The "positive" contrast bronchogram is seldom performed because patients [loved/hated] having thick oily goop dumped into their bronchi.

2

hated

Figure 7–2A shows a bronchogram with iodinated contrast outlining normal and dilated bronchi (bronchiectasis). Bronchography has been replaced by CT. Figure 7–2B shows mildly dilated bronchi *(arrows)* in otherwise normal right lung.

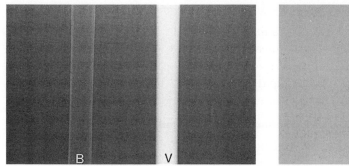

Figure 7–3A

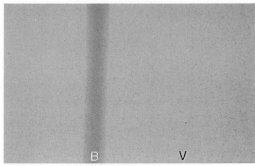

Figure 7–3B

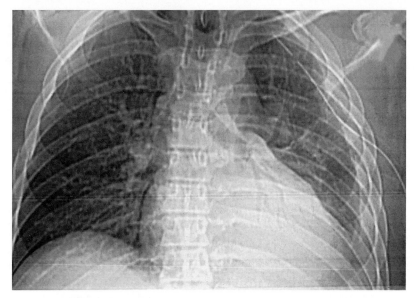

Figure 7–4

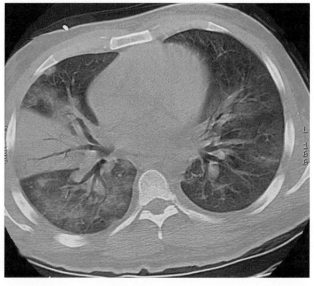

Figure 7–5

3

Do we ever see bronchi in the lung? Sure we do! When the lung is consolidated and the bronchi contain air, the dense lung delineates the air in the bronchi. Visualization of air in the *intrapulmonary* bronchi on a chest roentgenogram is called the **air bronchogram sign.** The presence of an air bronchogram is [normal/abnormal].

3

abnormal

4

Figure 7–3*A* portrays the normal lung. Straw V (vessel) contains water and straw B (bronchus) contains air. They are x-rayed in air. Straw _____ is easily seen. Straw _____ is much less visible because of _____ .

4

V
B
air inside and outside the thin-walled straw

5

Figure 7–3*B* portrays a diseased (consolidated) lung; the straws are immersed in water. Straw B is now _____ , the _____ sign.

Straw V now disappears, the _____ sign. If you missed this, review questions 1 to 4.

5

visible/air
bronchogram
silhouette

Figure 7–4 is a digital x-ray of a patient with LLL pneumonia. The bronchi appear as branching black tubes in the consolidated lung. In Figure 7–5, the CT shows an RML air bronchogram.*

---

*I don't Agree? Whatabout Silhouette sign (left heart border) indicating lingula involvement. What about fact that in 7-5 Anterior parts of lung not involved, why isn't this Anterior Basal seg of RLL. CR in (7-4) Is this a Big heart

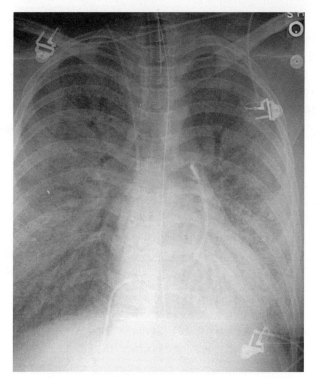

Figure 7–6

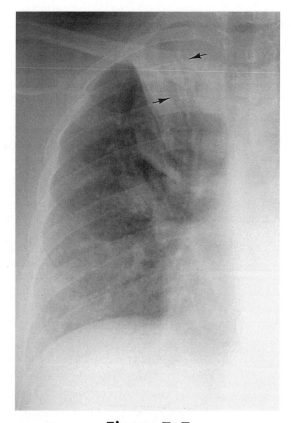

Figure 7–7

6

Soft tissue and air densities are involved in both the air bronchogram and silhouette signs. If an air-filled bronchus is to be seen, it must be surrounded by _____ density. Conversely, if a pulmonary vessel is to be seen, it must be surrounded by _____ .

6

soft tissue

air

Figure 7–6 is a patient with widespread airspace or alveolar consolidation. The bronchi are visible but the pulmonary vessels are not.

7

What good is the air bronchogram sign? Well, for one thing, bronchi are pulmonary structures; therefore, visualization of the bronchi (air bronchogram) denotes a _____ lesion and excludes a pleural or mediastinal lesion. It indicates that the bronchi contain _____ and the adjacent lung is _____ .

7

pulmonary

air
consolidated (radiodense)

Figure 7–7 shows a dense area of consolidation with air-filled bronchi *(arrows).* Because there is an air bronchogram sign, we know the lesion is in the lung and not in the mediastinum. Individual vessels are not visible because they are surrounded by water density.

8

The air bronchogram may be seen in pneumonia, pulmonary edema, pulmonary infarction, and certain chronic lung lesions. As long as the bronchi are _____ and the surrounding lung is radiopaque (water density), an _____ sign will be present.

8

air-filled

air bronchogram

In normal adults, only the trachea and main bronchi are visible. In normal *infants* and *young children,* the proximal portions of the lobar bronchi are often visible, as well.

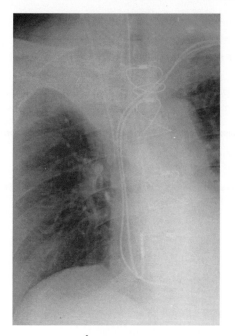

Figure 7–8

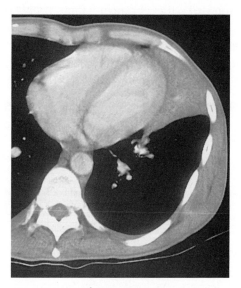

Figure 7–9

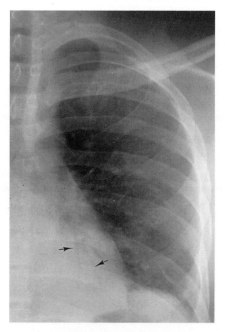

Figure 7–10

9

Do we always see an air bronchogram with pulmonary lesions? "Always", of course, is _____ the answer in medicine. If a bronchus is obstructed or filled with secretions, a pulmonary lesion (will/will not) show an air bronchogram.

9

never

will not

Patchy peripheral lung consolidation or interstitial disease usually does not cause an air bronchogram. Conditions that hyperinflate the lungs do not cause air bronchograms.

10

In pneumonia, if the bronchi are filled with secretions, there [will/will not] be an air bronchogram within the lesion. If a cancer obstructs a bronchus, an air bronchogram [will/will not] be visible. Interstitial edema [will/will not] cause an air bronchogram. Asthma [will/will not] cause an air bronchogram.

10

will not

will not/will not
will not

In Figure 7–8, there is no air bronchogram in the collapsed right upper lobe because the bronchi are full of mucous plugs. Compare with Figure 7–7. In Figure 7–9, there is no air bronchogram in the consolidated lingula because a tumor obstructs the proximal bronchus and the bronchial air has been replaced by secretions.

11

The presence of an air bronchogram indicates a _____ lesion. The *absence* of an air bronchogram indicates the lesion may be [pulmonary/extra pulmonary/either].

11

lung

either

Clinical Pearl: The heart shadow often obscures LLL disease. Sometimes an air bronchogram seen through the cardiac shadow is the most definitive sign of LLL consolidation. In Figure 7–10, air bronchograms *(arrows)* are visible through the density of the heart.

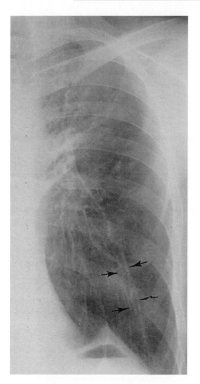

Figure 7–11

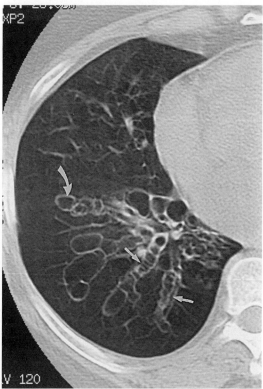

Figure 7–12

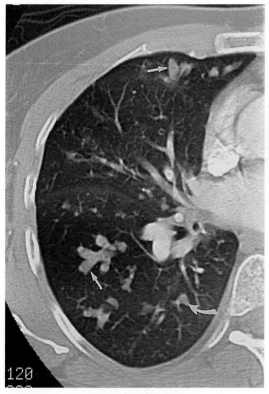

Figure 7–13

12

So far it's easy. But remember, consolidated lobes may *not* show an air bronchogram because the bronchi may be [*check correct answer(s)*]:
(a) filled with pus _____
(b) obstructed _____
(c) very thin-walled _____
(d) congenitally stenotic _____

12

✔*(a) filled with pus*
✔*(b) obstructed*
  (c) very thin-walled
✔*(d) congenitally stenotic*

Clinical Pearl: An air bronchogram indicates open airways, strong evidence that the lung disease is NOT due to an obstructing tumor.

13

Are there any other uses of the air bronchogram? If you see air-filled bronchi that are very crowded together, this is evidence of _____ of the lobe. The crowded air bronchograms suggest this is [obstructive/nonobstructive] atelectasis. In Figure 7–6, the bronchi are normally spaced, whereas in Figure 7–7, they are crowded (see p. 114).

13

collapse (atelectasis)
nonobstructive

14

Several diseases dilate the bronchi. Instead of tapering, the bronchi _____ as they course peripherally. This is termed "bronchiectasis."

14

widen (dilate)

Bronchiectasis is difficult to diagnose and illustrate on the x-ray. Figure 7–11 demonstrates dilated bronchi *(arrows)* with thickened walls. Figure 7–12 demonstrates dilated, thickened bronchi. Bronchi running in the axial plane are tubular *(arrows)* and bronchi running across the axial plane are circular *(curved arrow)*. Figure 7–13 demonstrates dilated bronchi completely filled with secretions both in plane *(arrows)* and in cross section *(curved arrow)*.

Anagram: Rearrange the letters in DORMITORY to form 2 words that better define it (answer on p. 121).

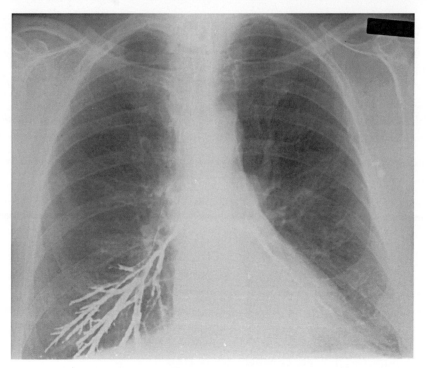

Figure 7–14

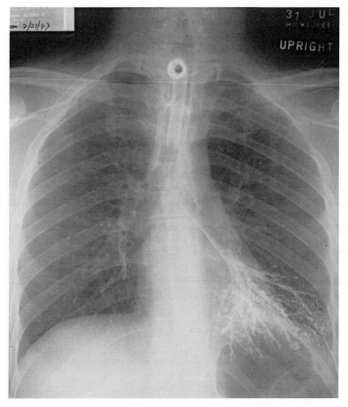

Figure 7–15

REVIEW

I

Any tubular structure (bronchus, vessel), viewed longitudinally, looks _____ . That same structure seen on end appears _____ . The inside of the bronchus is radiolucent because _____ , while the inside of a vessel is _____ because it contains blood.

I

linear
circular
it contains air
radiodense or radiopaque
(water density)

II

Which of the following conditions may show an air bronchogram?
(a) tuberculosis   (d) mediastinal bronchogenic cyst
(b) empyema   (e) bacterial pneumonia
(c) emphysema   (f) acute respiratory distress syndrome
                              (ARDS)

II

(a) tuberculosis
(e) bacterial pneumonia
(f) ARDS

III

A. Bronchi crowded together indicate _____ .
B. Dilated bronchi indicate _____ .
C. If an air bronchogram is visible, an endobronchial tumor is _____ .

III

A. collapse, atelectasis
B. bronchiectasis

C. very unlikely

IV

Figure 7–14 is that of an elderly patient and Figure 7–15 is that of a patient with a tracheostomy. Both have just finished a barium swallow.
A. What structures are outlined in white? _____
B. What anatomic areas are involved? _____
C. What is the white material and how did it get there? _____
D. Which patient has lower lobe atelectasis? _____

(Don't fret—aspirated barium is inert and is usually coughed up spontaneously.)

IV

A. bronchi
B. basal segments, lower lobes
C. aspirated barium

D. Figure 7–15, bronchi are close together

Anagram: Dormitory = Dirty Room

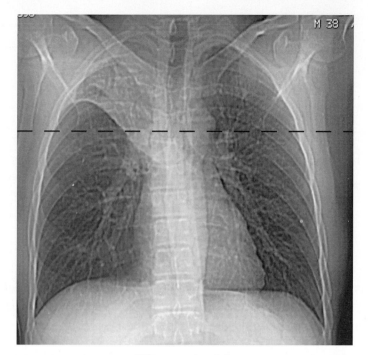

Figure 8–1A

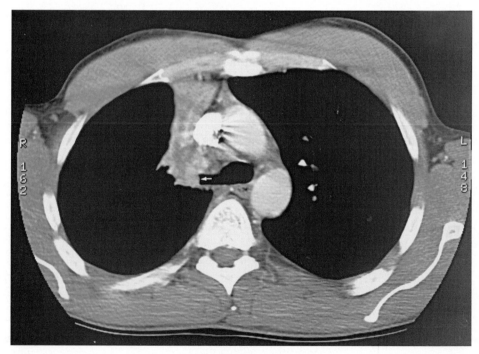

Figure 8–1B

Lobar and Segmental Collapse

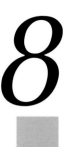

The lung has a natural tendency to collapse. Various physiologic mechanisms keep it expanded. When they fail, the lung loses volume. Now you can apply the radiographic anatomy you have learned to the subject of pulmonary collapse. In general, "collapse" describes severe volume loss and "atelectasis" describes mild or localized volume loss.

1

An abnormal lung, a lobe, or a segment may increase or decrease in size. *Collapse* or atelectasis obviously refers to a _____ in volume. There are four types of atelectasis: 1) resorption; 2) relaxation or passive; 3) cicatricial (scarring); and 4) adhesive. Hypoventilation also increases the tendency to lose volume.

2

If the airway is obstructed (e.g., a tumor or blood clot), air distal to the obstruction is _____ . Obstruction may be *central* (i.e., blocking a main, lobar, or segmental bronchus) or *peripheral* (i.e., blocking many small bronchi). Air distal to any _____ is *resorbed* and that portion of the lung _____ .

3

Central bronchial obstruction is caused by an intraluminal mass (intrinsic obstruction) or an extraluminal mass compressing a bronchus (extrinsic obstruction). Bronchogenic carcinoma is an example of _____ obstruction. A mediastinal tumor may cause _____ obstruction. Obstruction causes _____ atelectasis.

1

decrease

2

resorbed

obstruction
collapses (becomes atelectatic)

3

intrinsic
extrinsic
resorptive

Figure 8–1*A* is a PA digitized radiograph showing collapse of the RUL. In Figure 8–1*B*, a tumor *(arrow)* obstructs the RUL bronchus. Note the collapsed, airless lobe and the absence of air bronchograms.

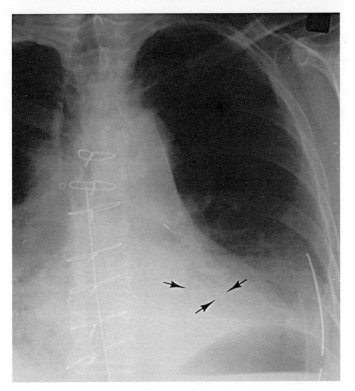

Figure 8–2

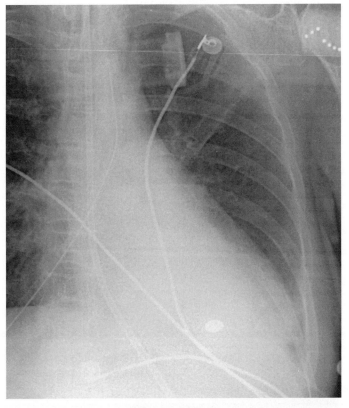

Figure 8–3

Clinical Pearl: In children, central obstruction is often due to a mucous plug or an aspirated foreign body. In adults under the age of 40, it is usually due to a mucous plug, a foreign body, or a benign tumor. In adults over the age of 40, bronchogenic carcinoma is a frequent cause of bronchial obstruction.

4

As a result of inflammatory exudate, mucus, hemorrhage, etc., many of the smaller bronchi may become plugged, resulting in [central/peripheral] obstructive collapse. The central bronchi should be [visible/invisible] on the radiograph.

4

peripheral
visible (contain air)

Figures 8–2 and 8–3 demonstrate postoperative lower lobe resorption atelectasis. Figure 8–2 shows peripheral obstructive atelectasis. The air bronchograms *(arrows)* indicate that lobar and segmental bronchi are open. Figure 8–3 shows central, obstructive atelectasis. The absence of air bronchograms indicates that the lobar bronchus is plugged with mucus. Postoperative hypoventilation undoubtedly contributes to the atelectasis.

5

The four mechanisms of collapse are 1) resorptive, 2) _____ , 3) _____ , and 4) _____ . A pneumothorax or pleural effusion separates the lung from the negative pressures generated by the chest wall and diaphragm during inspiration. The lung follows its natural tendency to _____ . This is _____ atelectasis.

5

relaxation (passive)/
adhesive/cicatricial

retract/relaxation (passive)

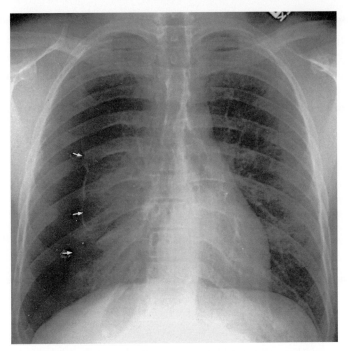

Figure 8–4

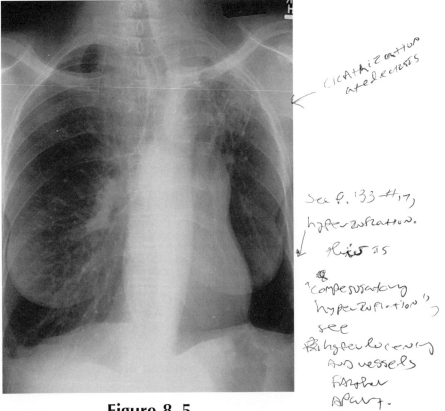

CICATRIZATION atelectases

See p. 133 #17, hyperinflation. this is "compensatory hyperinflation", see hyperlucency and vessels FArther APART.

Figure 8–5

Figure 8–4 shows collapse of the right lung due to a pneumothorax. The lung has been allowed to retract passively (*arrows* = edge of lung).

6

Pulmonary fibrosis, either local (e.g., tuberculous scarring, radiation fibrosis) or generalized, (e.g., silicosis, sarcoidosis), results in diminution in volume. This represents collapse from _____ .

6

cicatrization (scarring)

Figure 8–5 is a case of LUL cicatrization atelectasis caused by scarring from tuberculosis. The mediastinum is pulled toward the fibrosis.

7

Surfactant diminishes surface tension in the alveoli, helping the lung stay inflated. Diminished surfactant promotes volume loss. This is termed _____ atelectasis.

7

adhesive

Clinical Pearl: Respiratory distress syndrome of the newborn, acute respiratory distress syndrome, uremia, and cardiac bypass cause adhesive atelectasis from diminished surfactant.

8

State the mechanism of atelectasis for the conditions below:
(a) Bronchogenic carcinoma causes [intrinsic/extrinsic] obstruction, causing _____ atelectasis.
(b) Adenopathy from lymphoma causes [intrinsic/extrinsic] obstruction, causing _____ atelectasis.
(c) A hemothorax causes _____ atelectasis.
(d) Radiation fibrosis causes _____ atelectasis.

8

(a) intrinsic/resorptive

(b) extrinsic/resorptive

(c) relaxation (passive)
(d) cicatricial (contraction)

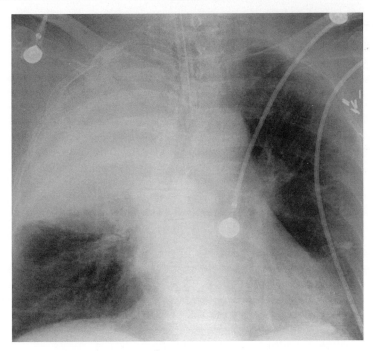

Figure 8–6

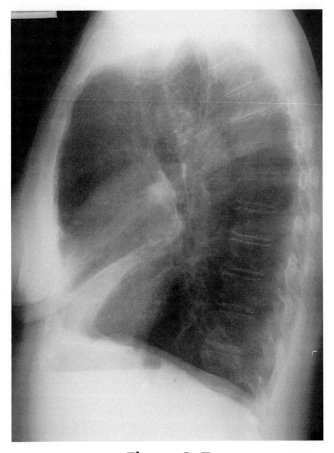

Figure 8–7

Hypoventilation worsens atelectasis, regardless of the primary mechanism. Is there anything that lessens or prevents atelectasis? If the lung parenchyma is very edematous or inflamed, or secretions can't drain past an obstruction, the lung will not collapse. Adhesions between the visceral and parietal pleura also prevent collapse. In Figure 8–6, tumor obstructs the RUL bronchus (no air bronchogram), but postobstructive pneumonia prevents collapse.

It is easy to recognize passive collapse by seeing the pneumothorax or the pleural fluid and cicatricial collapse by seeing irregular scarring in the collapsed lobe. Resorption collapse is often more difficult to diagnose. We must rely on other direct and indirect radiographic signs of atelectasis to make the diagnosis. *Direct* signs involve shift of adjacent fissures or lung marking in the affected lung. *Indirect* signs include shift of adjacent structures and changes in lung density.

9

If the volume of a lobe or segment is diminished, the adjacent fissure(s) will be displaced [toward/away from] the collapsed area. Figure 8–7 shows the minor fissure is displaced _____ and the major fissure is displaced _____ in RML collapse. When visible, shifting fissures are the most reliable *direct* radiographic sign of collapse.

9

toward

downward
forward (upward)

10

If a lobe or segment is atelectatic but still contains some air, the vascular markings will be visible but crowded into a [smaller/larger] space. If the bronchi are visible (the air bronchogram sign), they too will appear _____ together. Figure 8–2 (p. 124) shows crowded air bronchograms in LLL collapse.

10

smaller
crowded

11

If a "marker structure" (a nodule, granuloma, scar, surgical clip, etc.) shifts position in the atelectatic lung, it is a [direct/indirect] sign of volume loss.

11

direct

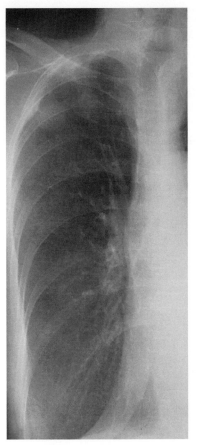

Figure 8–8A

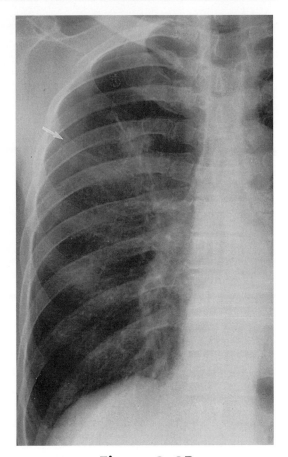

Figure 8–8B

Figure 8–8A demonstrates an RUL nodule. In Figure 8–8B, there is a pneumothorax following a needle biopsy. The pleural reflection or lung edge *(arrow)* is difficult to see, but the nodule has shifted centrally. (Yes, I did the biopsy.)

12

The three direct signs of collapse, then, are:

(1) _ø Shift of Adjacent fissuurs (most Reliable Direct sign)_

(2) _ø Shift of lung markings_

(3) _crowded bronchovascular markings_

12

(1) displaced fissure

(2) crowed bronchovascular markings

(3) shift of "marker" structures

13

Collapse may cause compensatory shift in adjacent structures, giving *indirect* signs of atelectasis. For example, if the right hilum shifts upward, there is collapse of the _____ . If the left hilum shifts downward, there is collapse of the _____ .

13

RUL

LLL

See page 135

For Indirect

Signs of collapse/atelectasis

Signs of At or collapse

Direct   Indirect

Shift of fissures   Structural shifts &

shift of lung
     markings
                     1. Hilum (most Reliable Indirect sign)

                     2. Diaphragm

                     3. Mediastinum

                     4. heart

                     5. Density

                        1. ↑'d opacity of collapsed lung

                        2. ↑'d lucency of over inflated lung
                           compensatory
                           hyperinflation

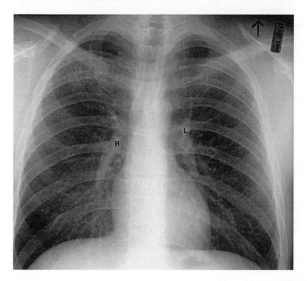

IN over 99%
left hilum is
higher than
the Right
IN 3% Equal

Figure 8–9A

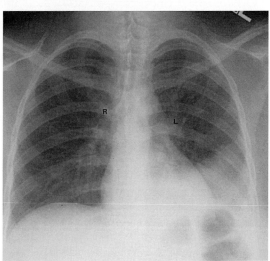

Figure 8–9B

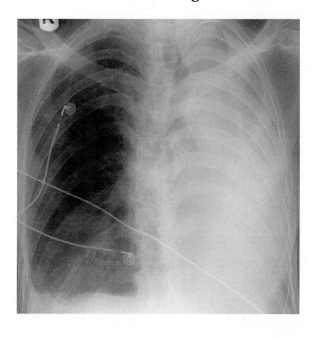

Figure 8–10

To appreciate hilar displacement one must know the relative positions of the normal hila. In over 97% of individuals, the left hilum (L) is slightly higher than the right (R) (see Fig. 8–9A). In the remaining 3%, the hila are at the same level. Figures are based on 1000 normal chest x-rays studied by Dr. Felson when he had nothing better to do (World War II—noncombat overseas assignment, wife in the US, and pretelevision).

14

Hilar depression indicates _____ collapse (Fig. 8–9B). Hilar elevation indicates _____ collapse (Fig. 8–1A, p. 122). Middle lobe and _____ atelectasis usually do not shift the hilum. Hilar shift is the most reliable _____ sign of atelectasis.

14

lower lobe

upper lobe

lingular

indirect

15

The other indirect signs rely on shift of structures [toward/ away from] the collapsed lung. For instance, in lobar atelectasis, the diaphragm is often [elevated/depressed]. This is a second *indirect* sign of volume loss. By the way, which diaphragm is usually higher? _____ (see Fig. 8–9A).

15

toward

elevated

the right, by a few cm

16

Similarly, mediastinal structures may shift. With upper lobe collapse, the trachea shifts [toward/away from] the lesion (Fig. 8–5, p. 126). With lower lobe collapse, the heart may shift [toward/away from] the side of collapse (Fig. 8–3, p. 124).

16

toward

toward

When a whole lung collapses, both the trachea and heart shift toward the lesion as in Figure 8–10.

17

Volume loss usually changes the density of the lung. The airless, atelectatic lung is [more/less] radiopaque. Adjacent lobes may hyperinflate to fill the void. This "compensatory hyperinflation" causes that area to be [more/less] radiolucent and the vessels to be [closer together/farther apart].

17

more

more
farther apart

Figure 8–10 shows increased lucency due to compensatory overinflation of the right lung. Figure 8–5 (p. 126) shows LLL hyperlucency due to compensatory hyperinflation for LUL collapse.

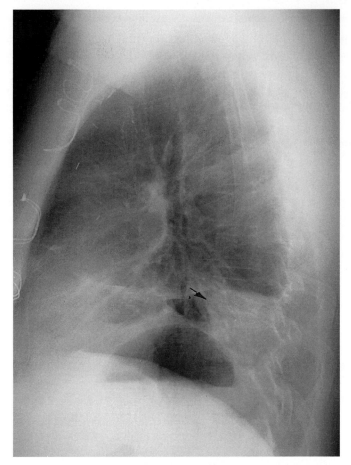

Figure 8–11A

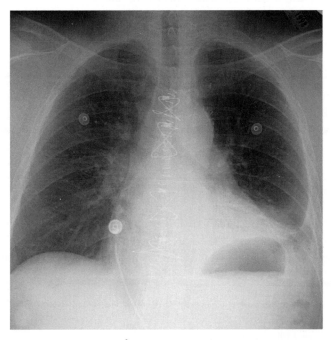

Figure 8–11B

18

Indirect signs of collapse include structural shifts and changing lung densities.

A. Name three structures that shift toward the lesion?

(1) _____   (3) _____

(2) _____

B. Name two structures that change density?

(1) _____   (2) _____

18

A. *(1) hilum*

    (2) diaphragm

    (3) mediastinum

B. *(1) collapsed lung, in-creased opacity*

    (2) overinflated lung, increased lucency

19

It is easy to apply these signs to specific lobes because the two lungs show similar signs of collapse. The RLL and LLL (and corresponding major fissures) collapse posteriorly, medially, and downward. On the lateral view, the major fissure is displaced [anteriorly/posteriorly] and [upward/downward]. On the frontal view, the lower lobe is radiodense and the hilum is _____ . On the right, the minor fissure is often [elevated/depressed] as the RML shifts downward to fill the void.

19

posteriorly

downward

low

depressed

Figure 8–11*A* shows that the major fissure *(arrow)* is posterior due to collapse of LLL basal segments. On the PA view, Figure 8–11*B*, the atelectatic basal segments are radiopaque. The hilum is low, the stomach bubble (diaphragm) is high, and the LUL is hyperlucent. Note a silhouette sign of the diaphragm on the PA and lateral film.

20

RML and lingula collapse are best seen on the lateral view because the x-ray beam is [parallel/perpendicular] to the flattened lobe (see Fig. 8–7, p. 128). In RML atelectasis, the minor fissure moves _____ and the lower part of the major fissure moves _____ . The middle lobe, between the fissures, is [radiolucent/radiodense].

20

parallel

downward

anteriorly

radiodense

Anagram: Twelve plus one =

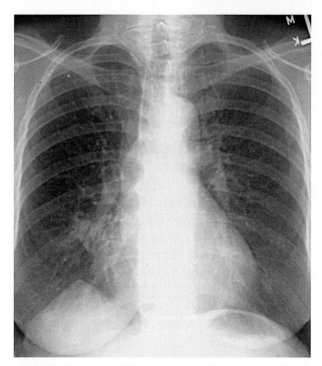

Figure 8–12A

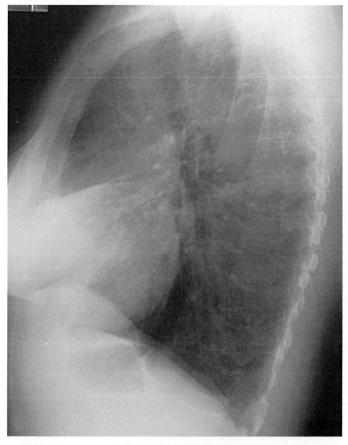

Figure 8–12B

21

The collapse of the RML and lingula often results in a vague increase in density on the frontal projection. The silhouette sign often comes to the rescue. Collapse of the RML obliterates the _____ and collapse of the lingula obliterates the _____ . The silhouette sign may be the only visible abnormality on the PA radiograph.

21

right heart border
left heart border

In Figure 8–12A, the collapsed RML is barely visible, but the right heart border shows a silhouette sign. In Figure 8–12B, the radiodense, flattened RML is easily seen on the lateral. The normal RML and lingula are small and atelectasis does not cause shifts of adjacent structures.

Clinical Pearl: The middle lobe is often slow to reinflate after collapse because it is compressed by the hyperinflated upper and lower lobes. The "RML syndrome" is a chronic nonobstructive atelectasis but it may mimic RML obstruction, radiographically.

22

Both upper lobes collapse in an upward, medial, and anterior direction. The upper portion of the major fissure moves [anteriorly/posteriorly]. With RUL atelectasis, the minor fissure moves [upward/downward] and [medially/laterally].

22

anteriorly
upward
medially

Anagram answer: Twelve plus one = eleven plus two

lower lobes collapse
posteriorly
medially
Downward

uppers collapse
Anteriorly
medially
upward

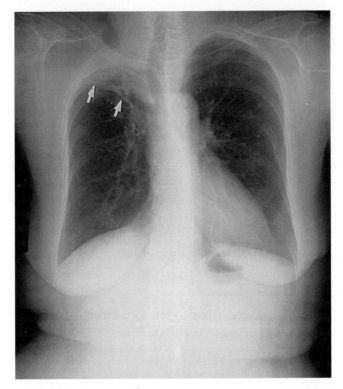

Figure 8–13

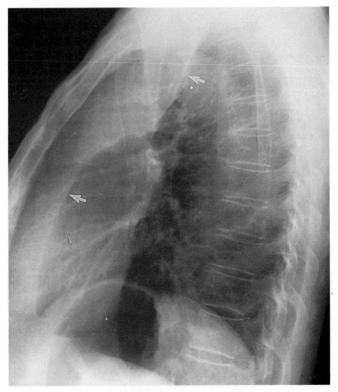

Figure 8–14A

23

Figure 8–13 shows RUL collapse with elevation and medial displacement of the minor fissure *(arrows)*. The right hilum is _____ and the trachea is _____ . If you missed this, you get the curse of the constipated termite—inability to pass boards.

23

elevated/shifted right

The superior and lingular divisions of the LUL often collapse as a unit since they share a common bronchus. In Figure 8–14A, the collapsed lobe moves forward. The major fissure *(arrows)* moves anteriorly. The hyperinflated lower lobe moves up and contacts the aortic arch. The expected silhouette sign of the aorta is absent on the PA film (Fig. 8–14B). Note the high diaphragm and hilum.

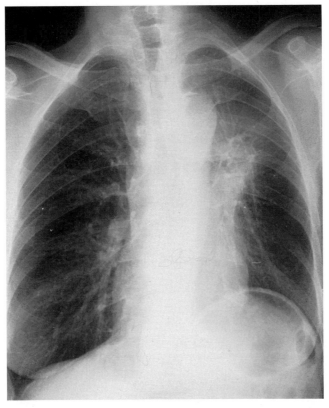

Figure 8–14B

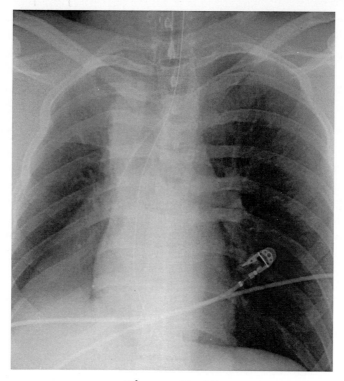

Figure 8–15

REVIEW

I

What is the principal mechanism of atelectasis for the following diseases?
(1) pleural effusion _____
(2) silicosis _____
(3) ARDS _____
(4) large hilar cancer _____

I

(1) relaxation (passive)
(2) cicatricial
(3) adhesive
(4) resorptive (obstructive, extrinsic)

II

Name the collapsed lobe(s):
(1) major fissure posterior, hilum down _____ or

_____

(2) minor fissure upward, major fissure anterior

_____

(3) hilum down, diaphragm up, heart border visible

_____

II

(1) RLL/LLL

(2) RUL

(3) RLL or LLL

III

Figure 8–15 is that of a patient 8 hours after general surgery. This is a chance for you to pull together what you have learned in the last several chapters.
A. Which lobes are collapsed? _____
B. Direct signs? _____
C. Indirect signs? _____
D. What are the most likely causes of the collapse in this situation? _____ and _____
E. Air bronchograms: [present/absent], indicating

_____
F. Silhouette sign: Where? _____

III

A. RUL, RLL
B. minor fissure up
C. mediastinal shift, diaphragm up, L hyperinflated, RUL, RLL radiopaque
D. resorption (retained secretions)/hypoventilation
E. absent/mucus in major bronchi
F. diaphragm, mediastinum

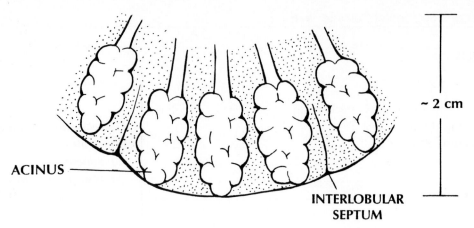

ACINUS

INTERLOBULAR
SEPTUM

~ 2 cm

Figure 9–1

Patterns of Lung Disease

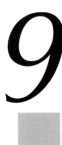

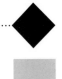

We have already seen how disease can consolidate or collapse a segment or lobe. We will now look at other patterns of diffuse and focal lung disease. The lung reacts to disease in a limited number of ways. The interstitium can thicken or thin and the alveoli can fill with fluid or extra air. These changes may be focal or diffuse. They may be acute or chronic. This leads to 16 possible combinations: (interstitium = thick/thin) × (alveoli = fluid/air) × (location = focal/diffuse) × (time = acute/chronic). Relax. We will concentrate only on the most common combinations. These four basic variables will help us analyze the chest x-ray and form a differential diagnosis.

1

First, a brief review. For each chest radiograph, we ask, *"Are There Many Lung Lesions?"*

A = _____   L = _____
T = _____   L = _____
M = _____

Review the search patterns outlined in Figure 3–5 through Figure 3–8 (pp. 44–50), if necessary.

1

abdomen
thorax (bones and soft tissue)
mediastinum
lung—unilateral
lung—bilateral

2

Conceptually, the lung has two components, the supporting structures (arteries, veins, bronchi, etc.), known as the _____ , and the air sacs, known as the _____ . Air sacs form acini and several acini form a _____ . Review Figure 9–1.

2

interstitium
alveoli
secondary pulmonary lobule

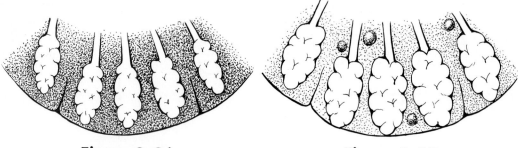

Figure 9–2A   **Figure 9–2B**

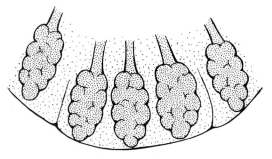

Figure 9–2C

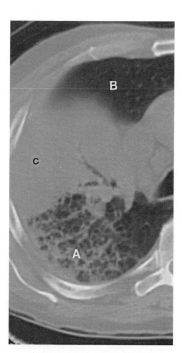

Figure 9–3A

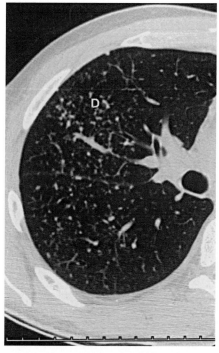

Figure 9–3B

3

On a chest x-ray, the visible "interstitium" is basically the branching _____ . As they branch, they disappear peripherally because they are _____ .

pulmonary vessels beyond the resolution of the x-ray

4

The air-filled alveoli are too small to resolve, but in total they appear uniformly [radiolucent/radiodense].

radiolucent

Most lung diseases result in increased radiodensity of the lung. If the interstitium thickens, it can be seen more peripherally on the x-ray or CT. If the interstitial thickening is generalized, the pattern is linear (reticular) (Fig. 9–2A). If the thickening is discrete, it forms multiple, tiny nodules (Fig. 9–2B). If the alveoli fill with fluid, the fluid-filled area becomes radiodense and the interstitium is enveloped in the density (Fig. 9–2C).

5

Match the descriptions below with the CT patterns shown in Figure 9–3A and B.
(1) normal _____
(2) alveolar filling disease _____
(3) linear (reticular) interstitial thickening _____
(4) nodular interstitial thickening _____

5

B
C
A
D

In your mind's eye (whatever that is), fuse the patterns in Figure 9–2 with those in Figure 9–3.

INterstitium
thick
a
thin

alveoli
fluid
or
Air

location
focal
a
diffuse

time
chronic
a
Acute

linear = Reticular

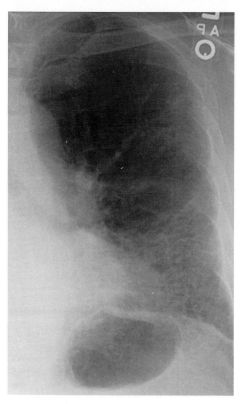

Figure 9–4A

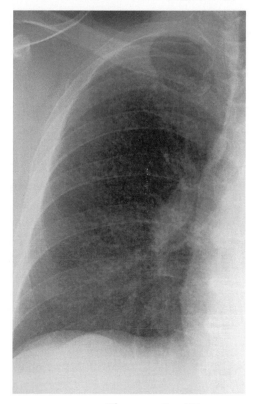

Figure 9–4B

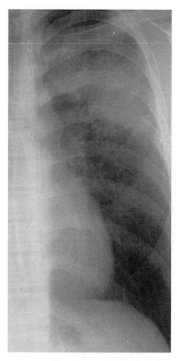

Figure 9–4C

6

Match the patterns listed below with the patterns illustrated in Figure 9–4A, B, and C.

(1) alveolar filling disease _____

(2) reticular (linear) interstitial thickening _____

(3) nodular interstitial thickening

_____

6

(1) Figure 9–4C

(2) Figure 9–4A

(3) Figure 9–4B

7

Let's look at the specific patterns. In *interstitial lung disease,* the peribronchovascular tissue thickens. This makes the vessels or "markings" appear [more/less] prominent. At the same time, the alveoli are still _____ . The basic appearance is one of aerated lung but too many "markings."

7

more
aerated

Clinical Pearl: Frequent causes of interstitial thickening include edema, inflammation, tumor, and fibrosis.

8

Figure 9–4A and B demonstrates prominent interstitial markings, which may be in one area of the lung (focal) or generalized (diffuse).

1. In Figure 9–4A, the dominant pattern is (linear/nodular) and (diffuse/focal).

2. In Figure 9–4B, the dominant pattern is (linear/nodular) and (diffuse/focal).

8

linear
focal
nodular
diffuse

9

In general, *acute* and *chronic* interstitial lung disease looks similar. If the markings are hazy (ill-defined) and not distorted (i.e., normal branching pattern), the disease is probably [acute/chronic]. If the lung markings are sharp (well-defined) and distorted (i.e., angular, irregular branching), the disease is probably [acute/chronic].

9

acute

chronic

Clinical Pearl: The most reliable method of distinguishing acute from chronic is by viewing past films or, heaven forbid, taking a history. This is not cheating. It is synthesizing information to arrive at the best possible answer for the patient.

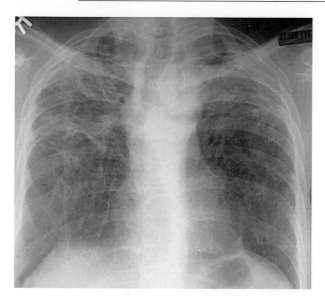

Figure 9–5A

Chronic
Interstitial
lung dz
Markings – Distorted
and distinct (sharp)

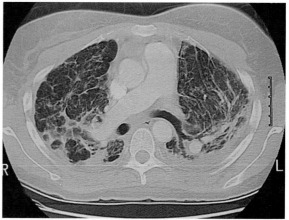

Figure 9–5B

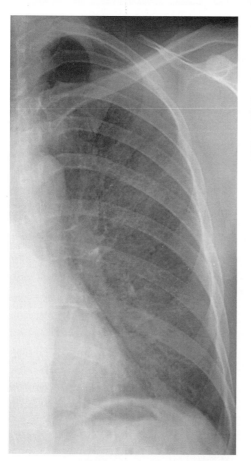

Figure 9–6

Acute interstitial lung dz
Markings – Not distorted
hazy

10

In Figure 9–5A, there is diffuse interstitial lung disease. The "interstitial" markings are [increased/decreased], while the alveoli are [aerated/airless]. It is chronic because the markings are [distorted/not distorted] and [distinct/indistinct]. In Figure 9–5B, the CT shows distorted and sharp interstitium and aerated lung.

increased
aerated
distorted
distinct

11

In Figure 9–6 the interstitial markings are increased. The margins are [sharp/hazy] and the markings are [distorted/not distorted]. This suggests [acute/chronic] disease. Compare with Figure 9–5A.

hazy
not distorted
acute

Clinical Pearl: Most diffuse interstitial lung disease is chronic and usually due to fibrosis. Acute diffuse interstitial lung disease is usually due to pulmonary edema and viral/mycoplasma pneumonia.

12

Match the patterns in the first column with the likely cause in the second column:

1. Interstitial markings are thickened.

   _____

2. Interstitial markings are very sharp.

   _____

3. Interstitial markings are indistinct.

   _____

4. Interstitial markings are distorted.

   _____

5. Interstitial markings change over several days. _____

(A) acute

(B) chronic

(C) acute or chronic

   _____

12

1 = C

2 = B

3 = A

4 = B

5 = A

We have just learned that the majority of diffuse *interstitial* lung disease is chronic. The majority of *alveolar disease* (airspace consolidation), whether *focal, multifocal,* or *diffuse,* is acute. With alveolar disease, the airspaces are filled with fluid (edema, blood, mucus, etc.), making the lung appear airless (radiodense, opaque, consolidated). The alveolar pattern may be relatively homogeneous (a lobe or segment) or patchy and scattered throughout the lung.

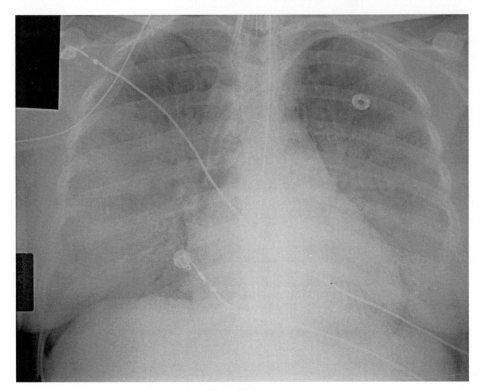

Figure 9–7

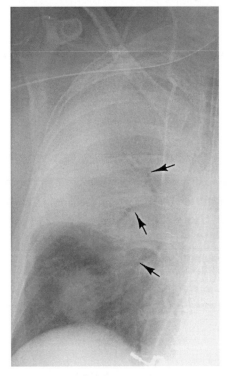

Figure 9–8

13

In Figure 9–7, there is *diffuse* [alveolar/interstitial] disease. The interstitial markings [are/are not] visible within the consolidated areas. This concept is similar to the _____ sign, because water density lung is in direct contact with the water density pulmonary vessels (interstitium).

14

Alveolar consolidation will cause a silhouette sign with the diaphragm, heart, or aorta only if _____. The silhouette sign is usually [present/absent] in interstitial disease because _____ is adjacent to these structures.

15

The air bronchogram (remember the air bronchogram?) is usually seen in [alveolar/interstitial] disease because the major airways are [open/plugged] but surrounded by consolidated (water density) lung. In interstitial disease, the bronchi are still surrounded by _____ .

13
alveolar
are not

silhouette

14

indirect contact
absent
aerated lung

15

alveolar
open

aerated lung

Figure 9–8 shows airspace consolidation of the RUL, an air bronchogram *(arrows)*, and a silhouette sign of the upper heart and mediastinum—three important signs of alveolar filling disease. There is also focal consolidation of the RLL without an air bronchogram or silhouette sign.

16

An air bronchogram means the bronchus contains _____ but is surrounded by [alveolar infiltrate/ aerated lung]. However, if mucus or other fluid fills the bronchi, the air bronchogram will be [absent/present] even in the face of adjacent airspace consolidation.

16
air
alveolar infiltrate

absent

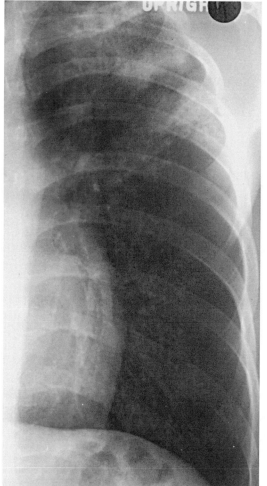

Figure 9–9

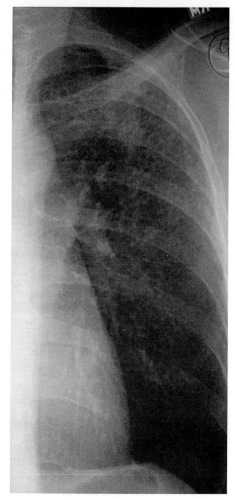

Figure 9–10A

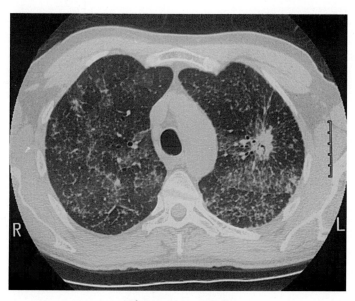

Figure 9–10B

17

To recap:

A. The air bronchogram and silhouette signs are often present with _____ .

B. However, with alveolar consolidation, the air bronchogram will be absent if _____ .

C. With alveolar consolidation, the silhouette sign will be absent if _____ .

17

A. *alveolar (airspace) consolidation*
B. *fluid fills the bronchi*
C. *not in direct contact with water density structure*

Clinical Pearl: The most frequent causes of diffuse alveolar disease (airspace filling disease) are bacterial pneumonia and severe pulmonary edema. The most frequent cause of acute focal alveolar consolidation is also infection.

18

Figure 9–9 is an example of multi *focal* alveolar disease. Within the consolidation, the interstitial markings are [visible/not visible]. Air bronchograms are more frequently absent in [central/peripheral] airspace consolidation. The age of the lesion is most accurately assessed with _____ . History is helpful but less reliable.

18

not visible

peripheral

old radiographs

To make life difficult, some diseases have both alveolar consolidation and interstitial thickening. Figure 9–10A shows focal LUL alveolar consolidation and diffuse interstitial thickening. Figure 9–10B demonstrates the two patterns nicely.

An important form of focal alveolar disease is the mass or nodule (the famous "spot on the lung"). If a very focal consolidate has well-defined borders and measures greater than 3 cm, it is referred to as a "mass." If it is less than 3 cm, it is called a "nodule."

Focal consolidate
c̄ well-defined
Borders
>3cm = MASS
<3cm = nodule

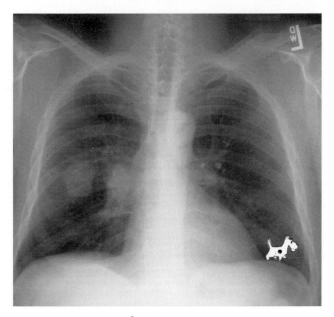

Figure 9–11

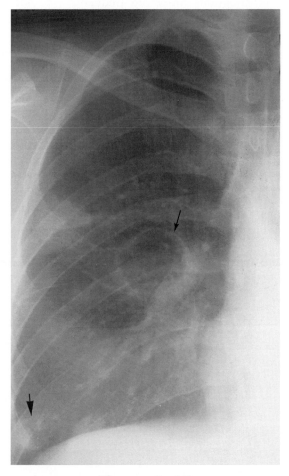

Figure 9–12

19

In Figure 9–11, there is a focal [alveolar/interstitial] opacity on the right. It has distinct margins and measures over 3 cm. It is termed a _____ . If it measured 1.5 cm, it would be termed a _____ . In the LLL is another _____ .

19

alveolar

mass
nodule
spot on the lung*

Clinical Pearl: Chronic alveolar infiltrates, nodules, and masses are most often due to indolent infection or inflammatory lung disease. Over the age of 40, cancer becomes a major concern.

20

When any alveolar lesion (infiltrate, mass, nodule) becomes necrotic, the liquefied material is usually expectorated and replaced with _____ . The center of the cavity becomes [radiodense/radiolucent].

20

air
radiolucent

Figure 9–12 demonstrates multiple masses, two of which are cavitary *(arrows)*.

---

*This is the "spot on the lung" patients often talk about.

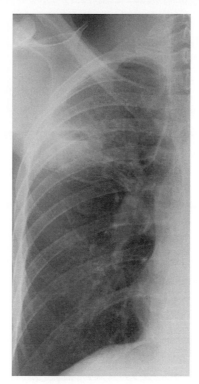

Figure 9–13

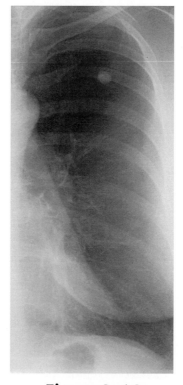

Figure 9–14

21

If the necrotic material is only partially expelled, an _____ / _____ level is formed. This is visible only when the x-ray beam is [parallel/perpendicular] to the interface. An air/fluid level is seen only in [erect/supine] frontal radiographs.

21

air/fluid
parallel

erect

Figure 9–13 demonstrates an air/fluid level in a cavitary RUL pneumonia. Compare with Figure 9–12, where there is no fluid in the cavities.

22

If caseous material is not expelled, it may heal and organize into a granuloma (a scar). Granulomas frequently calcify. Figure 9–14 shows a nodule in the LUL. It is [denser/less dense] than the rib, therefore it is _____ . This is most likely a [healed scar/cancer].

22

denser
calcified
healed scar

Clinical Pearl: Heavy calcification is an important sign of benign disease in the lung. Healed TB and histoplasmosis are the most frequent causes of lung granulomas.

GRANULOMAS

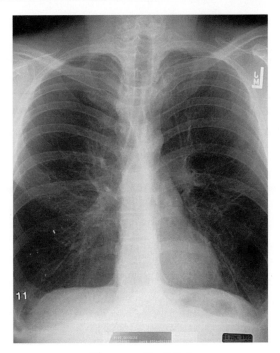

Figure 9–15A

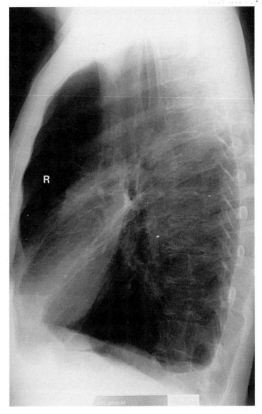

Figure 9–15B

Few conditions cause the lung to be more radiolucent. If the lung is hyperinflated, it becomes hyperlucent because a fixed amount of tissue is spread over a larger volume. If the interstitium is destroyed (i.e., bulla formation), the lung becomes hyperlucent because there is less tissue to absorb radiation. Bullae or sparse markings replace or distort normal branching vessels (Figs. 9–15, 9–16).

23

The combination of hyperinflation and _____ indicates emphysema. On the frontal view, diaphragmatic changes indicate hyperinflation. In Figure 9–15*A*, the diaphragms are flat and [normal/elevated/depressed]. They are lower than the _____ posterior rib. The diaphragms are normally at the ninth or tenth posterior rib.

23

bullae (sparse or distorted markings)

depressed
eleventh

24

Hyperinflation is also seen on the lateral. In Figure 9–15*B*, the sternum is [normal/bowed/sunken]. The "retrosternal clear space," the area between the ascending aorta and the sternum (R), is [normal/increased/decreased]. The diaphragms are _____ , and _____ . The AP diameter is increased (barrel chest).

24

bowed

increased
flat/depressed

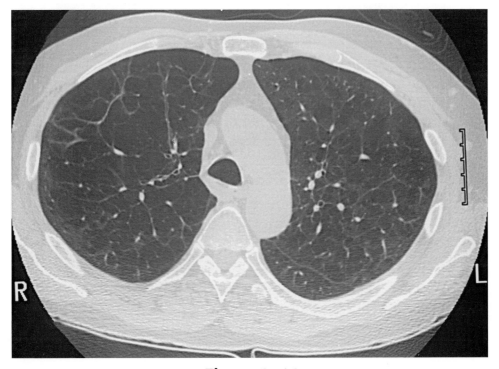

Figure 9–16

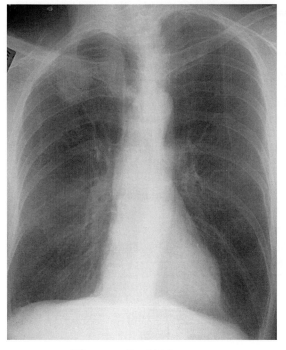

Figure 9–17A

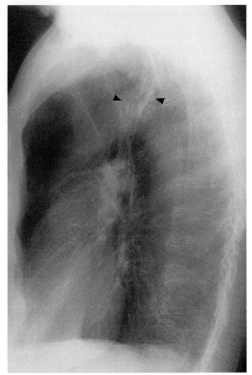

Figure 9–17B

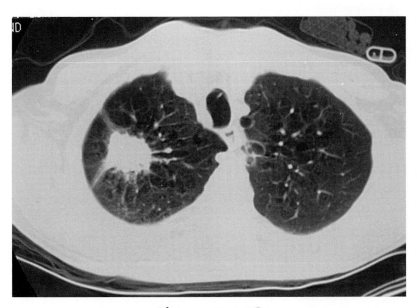

Figure 9–17C

REVIEW

I

Radiologic signs of diffuse *interstitial* lung disease:
1. "Pulmonary markings" are [more/less] visible.
2. The lung appears [aerated/not aerated].
3. An air bronchogram is [often/seldom] visible.
4. The silhouette sign [is/is not/may be] visible.
5. Acute disease causes [distortion/no distortion] of lung pattern.

I

1—more
2—aerated
3—seldom
4—is not
5—no distortion

II

Radiographic signs of *alveolar* filling disease or airspace consolidation:
1. Vessels are [more/less] visible in the area of disease.
2. The diseased lung appears [aerated/not aerated].
3. An air bronchogram [is/is not/may be] visible.
4. A silhouette sign [is/is not/may be] visible.

II

1. less
2. not aerated
3. may be
4. may be

III

In Figure 9–17*A* and *B:*
1. The patient has what generalized lung disease?
   _____
2. There is a focal _____ in the _____ lobe, _____ segment.
3. He has had one too many [drinks/cigarettes/lovers].
4. On Figure 9–17C, how does CT confirm your suspicions? _____

III

1. COPD (emphysema)
2. mass/RUL/posterior

3. cigarettes
4. RUL mass, emphysema, cigarettes and lighter in left breast pocket

---

In real life, these nice, neat patterns of lung disease often overlap. However, this approach provides a way of organizing your descriptions to form a differential diagnosis.

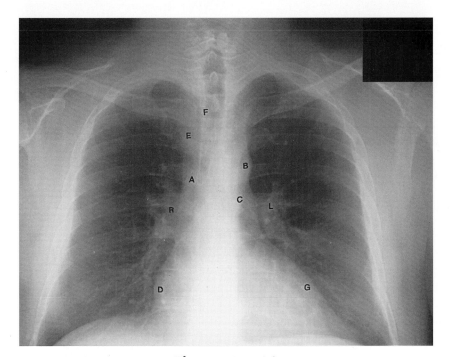

Figure 10–1A

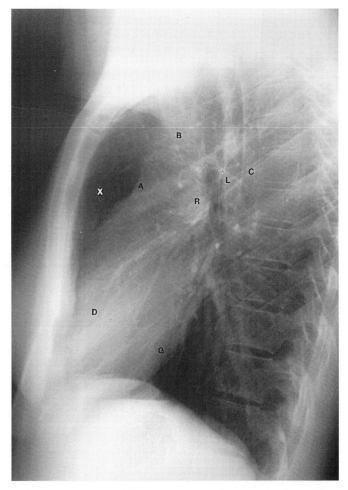

Figure 10–1B

The Mediastinum

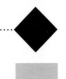

The mediastinum is the area between the right and left lungs, bounded by the medial parietal pleura. Mediastinal diseases can be difficult to detect on the chest x-ray because most are of soft tissue density and are surrounded by soft tissue structures. Mediastinal lesions may cause local or diffuse widening; displace, compress, or invade adjacent structures; or cause a silhouette sign with adjacent structures.

1

Let's review the mediastinal borders. On Figure 10–1A, identify the following:

A. _____   E. _____
B. _____   F. _____
C. _____   G. _____
D. _____

(The left and right pulmonary arteries [L and R], which define the hilum, are outside the mediastinum, in the lung.)

2

There is considerable overlap of the mediastinal structures in the PA view. The lateral view is often helpful for localization. In Figure 10–1B, identify the following:

A. _____   G. _____
B. _____   L. _____
C. _____   R. _____
D. _____

The lucent area (X) between the sternum and the ascending aorta is called the _____ .

3

The mediastinum completely separates the left and right pleural spaces in every animal but the _____ .
("Man is the missing link between animals and human beings." Konrad Lorenz)

1

A. *ascending aorta*
B. *aortic knob (arch)*
C. *descending aorta*
D. *right heart*
E. *superior vena cava*
F. *right tracheal wall*
G. *left heart*

2

A. *ascending aorta*
B. *aortic knob*
C. *descending aorta*
D. *right heart*
G. *left heart*
L. *left pulmonary artery*
R. *right pulmonary artery*
X. *retrosternal clear space*

3

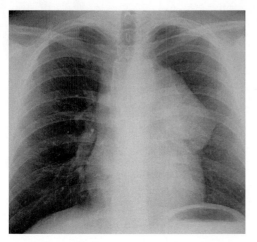

Figure 10–2A

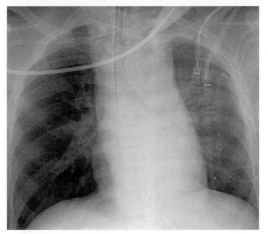

Figure 10–2B

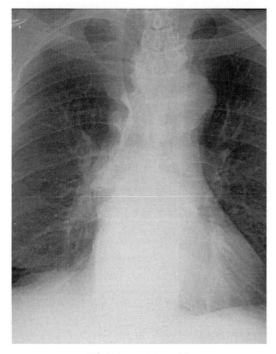

Figure 10–3A

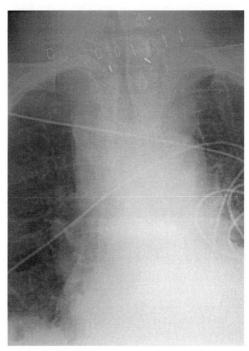

Figure 10–3B

4

The most frequent sign of mediastinal disease is mediastinal widening. Most masses cause [focal/generalized] widening, while infiltrating diseases (hemorrhage, infection, or tumor) usually cause [focal/generalized] widening.

4

focal

generalized

5

Figure 10–2A and B shows two cases of mediastinal disease. Which is likely due to tumor? _____
Why? _____
Which is likely due to hemorrhage? _____
Why? _____

5

Figure 10–2A
tumor, focal
Figure 10–2B
hemorrhage, diffuse

6

The bulging mediastinum displaces the mediastinal (medial parietal) pleura toward the lung. Therefore, the interface with the lung is usually [sharp/unsharp] and [concave/convex].

6

sharp
convex

7

Masses in an enclosed space may also displace, compress, or invade adjacent structures. In Figure 10–3A, the trachea is [midline/displaced] but its lumen is open. In Figure 10–3B, the trachea is [midline/displaced] but the lumen is _____ .

7

displaced
midline
narrowed (compressed)

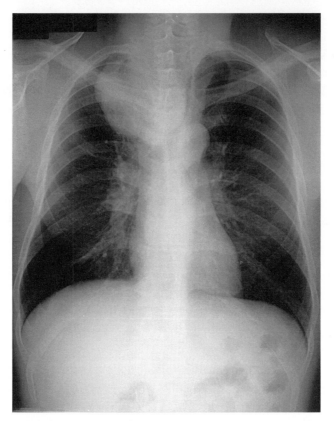

Figure 10–4

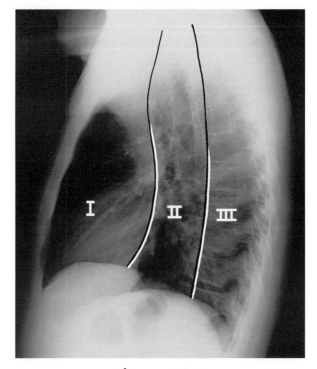

Figure 10–5

8

Finally, a mediastinal mass may obscure an adjacent structure of the same density, the _____ sign. This
helps to locate the mass. Figure 10–4 shows a large mass
obliterating the _____ border. Since the trachea
is in the middle mediastinum, this is a _____
mediastinal mass. Note tracheal displacement and nar-
rowing.

8

silhouette

*right tracheal (right medi-
astinal)*
middle

9

A review:
(1) Most mediastinal masses cause a _____ widening of the mediastinum.
(2) Most mediastinal infiltration (blood, infection) will
cause a _____ widening of the mediastinum.
(3) In both cases, the interface with the lung is usually _____ and _____ .
(4) Secondary signs of mediastinal disease include inva-
sion, _____ , _____ , and a
_____ sign.

9

(1) focal

(2) diffuse

(3) sharp/convex

*(4) displacement/com-
pression/silhouette*

For convenience of differential diagnosis, the mediastinum is divided into three
compartments: anterior, middle, and posterior. There are several methods of dividing the mediastinum. None is perfect because structures and diseases often cross
these artificial divisions. Felson's is the simplest (and we like simple). ("Get the
facts first, then distort them as you please." Mark Twain)

10

The radiologist divides the mediastinum into three compartments based on the lateral chest x-ray. In Figure 10–5,
an imaginary line separates the anterior (I) and middle (II)
mediastinum. It sits in front of the trachea but behind
the _____ . A line, 1 cm back from the anterior
edge of the vertebral bodies, separates the _____
mediastinum from the _____ mediastinum (III).

10

heart
middle
posterior

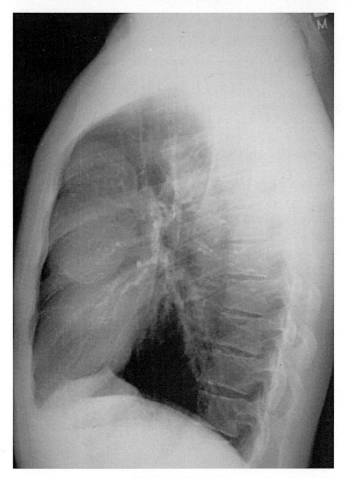

Figure 10–6

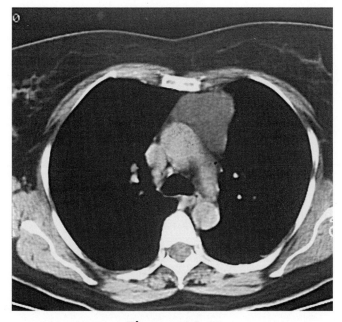

Figure 10–7

11

The anterior mediastinal compartment sits between the sternum and a line drawn anterior to the _____ and posterior to the _____ . On the lateral x-ray, this is the retrosternal clear space.

12

The lateral radiograph is often helpful in assigning disease to one of the mediastinal compartments. In Figure 10–6, the mass sits in the _____ mediastinum. It fills the retrosternal clear space.

13

What lesions cause anterior mediastinal masses? "Snow White and the Seven Dwarfs" dwell in the forest. "Big White and the Five T's" dwell in the anterior mediastinum. Big White is the _____ and the five T's are named Thyroid, Thymus, Teratoma, Thoracic aorta (ascending), and Terrible lymphoma. (Big White is discussed in Chapter 12.)

11

trachea
heart

12

anterior

13

heart

> Bis white
> +
> 5 T's dwell
> Anterior:
> heart
> Thyroid
> Thymus
> Thoracic Aorta
> terrible lymphoma
> teratoma

In Figure 10–2A and Figure 10–6, the patients have thymic masses. In general, it is difficult to differentiate one anterior mediastinal mass from another on the chest x-ray. CT is often helpful. In Figure 10–7, the CT shows a homogeneous anterior mediastinal mass with sharp margins, filling the clear space. It is also a thymoma.

14

The middle mediastinum is located between a line anterior to the _____ , posterior to the _____ , and a line _____ .

15

Which of the following structures are located in the middle mediastinum?

A. esophagus _____ E. thymus _____
B. heart _____ F. aortic arch _____
C. lymph nodes _____ G. ascending aorta _____
D. trachea _____

14

trachea/heart/1 cm behind anterior edge of vertebral bodies

15

> Middle mediastinum

A. esophagus
C. lymph nodes
D. trachea
F. aortic arch

Clinical Pearl: Enlarged lymph nodes are the most frequent cause of a middle mediastinal mass.

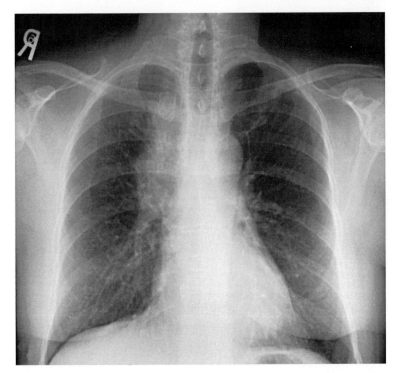

Figure 10–8A

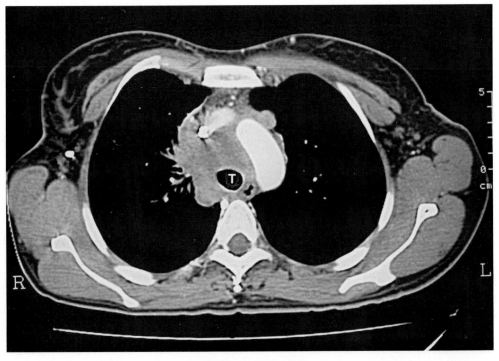

Figure 10–8B

16

In Figure 10–8*A*, there is a lobulated mass obscuring the right tracheal border. The trachea is located in the _____ mediastinum. This is a _____ mediastinal mass. The mass is _____ toward the lung and is lobulated but has sharp borders.

16

middle/middle

convex

Figure 10–8*B* is a CT demonstrating the enlarged lymph nodes to the right of and anterior to the trachea (T) in the middle mediastinum. NOTE: The nodes prevent the lung from contacting the right tracheal wall.

17

Most midmediastinal lesions arise from the _____ . The other three major middle mediastinal organs are the _____ , _____ , and the _____ .

17

lymph nodes

esophagus/trachea/aorta (arch and descending)

Anagram: mother-in-law

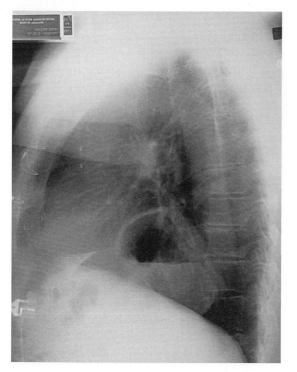

Figure 10–9A

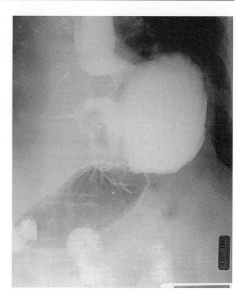

Figure 10–9B

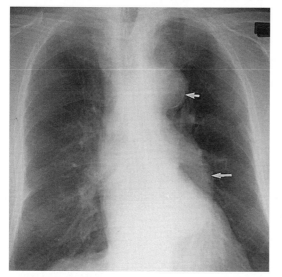

Figure 10–10A

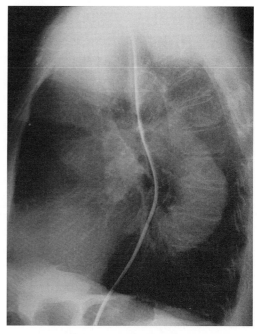

Figure 10–10B

18

Study Figure 10–9A. There is a mass in the _____ mediastinum. What unusual feature is present? _____ . This suggests the lesion is in the esophagus.

19

In the middle mediastinum, if one suspects an esophageal lesion, the appropriate exam would be a _____ . If one suspects a solid tumor, adenopathy, or a tracheal lesion, the appropriate exam would be a _____ . Figure 10–9B is an anteroposterior barium swallow (esophagram) showing a large hiatal hernia (stomach above diaphragm).

18

middle

air/fluid level

19

barium swallow

CT

Primary tracheal lesions are rare, but keep your eye on the trachea because it is often deviated or narrowed by adjacent lesions.

20

Don't forget that vascular structures also traverse the mediastinum. The ascending aorta is in the [anterior/middle/posterior] mediastinum on the right and the aortic arch is in the [anterior/middle/posterior] mediastinum as it crosses from right to left. In Felson's classification, the descending aorta is a _____ mediastinal structure. As it elongates with age, it usually overlaps the spine.

20

anterior

middle

posterior

In Figure 10–10A, an aneurysmal aortic arch projects as a mass. Note the calcified (atherosclerotic) intima *(short arrow)*. The tortuous descending aorta is lateral to the heart *(long arrow)*. Figure 10–10B shows the tortuous descending aorta overlapping the spine. A feeding tube demonstrates the course of the esophagus, a middle mediastinal structure.

Anagram answer: Woman Hitler

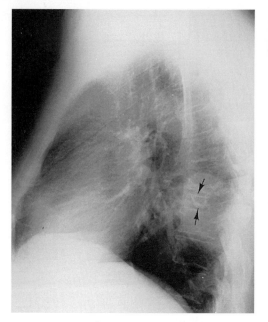

Figure 10–11A

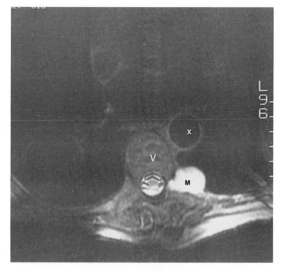

Figure 10–11B

Figure 10–12

21

Which structures are located in the posterior mediastinum?

A. esophagus   _____   D. vertebral bodies_____

B. lymph nodes   _____   E. descending aorta_____

C. spinal nerves _____

21   *Posterior mediastinum*

B. lymph nodes

C. spinal nerves

D. vertebral bodies

E. descending aorta

22

The posterior mediastinum sits between a line _____ and the posterior ribs. More simply, the posterior mediastinum is the paravertebral area.

22

1 cm behind anterior edge of the vertebral bodies

23

In Figure 10–11A, a large mass overlies the spine. It may be in the lung or in the _____ . The arrows point to a destroyed and collapsed vertebral body, suggesting that this mass is in the _____ . Figure 10–11B demonstrates multiple myeloma of the vertebral body producing the paraspinous mass and destroying the vertebral body and adjacent rib.

23

posterior mediastinum

posterior mediastinum

Figure 10–12; an MRI, shows a neural tumor. The vertebral body (V) is intact but a soft tissue mass (M) protrudes through the neural foramen into the posterior mediastinum. The descending aorta (x) is normal.

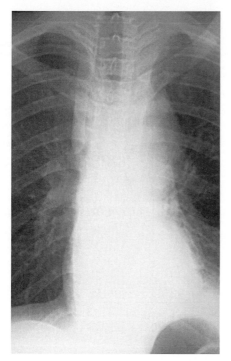

Figure 10–13A

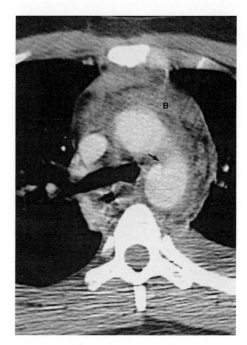

Figure 10–13B

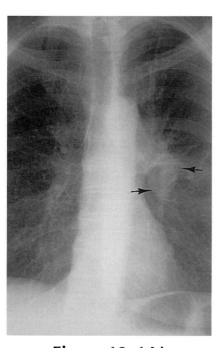

Figure 10–14A

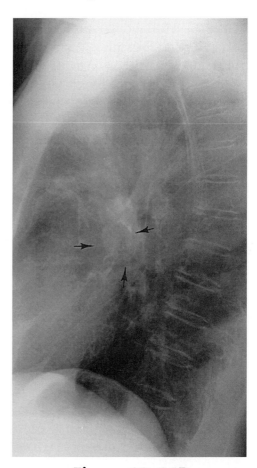

Figure 10–14B

Clinical Pearl: Most posterior mediastinal masses are from the nerves or their coverings (neurofibroma, meningocele, etc.) in younger patients. Aortic aneurysms, multiple myeloma, and metastatic spine diseases are more common in older patients.

24

Infection, hemorrhage, adenopathy, and infiltrating tumor may involve several mediastinal compartments. This usually causes a [focal/generalized] mediastinal widening.

24

generalized

In Figure 10–13A, there is diffuse widening of the mediastinum after trauma. In Figure 10–13B, the CT shows blood (B) in the mediastinum. The descending aorta is irregular *(arrow)* due to a posttraumatic laceration of the aorta. Did you see the LLL collapse on Figure 10–13A?

25

The mediastinum sits [central/lateral] to the medial parietal pleura. The hilum sit [central/lateral] to the medial parietal. On the chest x-ray, the visible structures we call the hilum are the _____ . They taper as they course inferiorly.

25

central
lateral

pulmonary vessels

The most common cause of a hilar mass is adenopathy or an adjacent tumor. In Figure 10–14A, the normal right hilum gets thinner inferiorly. The left hilum gets wider because of a left hilar tumor *(arrows)*. Figure 10–14B shows the tumor on the lateral *(arrows)*.

The chest x-ray is reasonably sensitive in detecting mediastinal lesions. Additional imaging is usually required to characterize the abnormality. This is where your clinical understanding and the patient's history and physical findings define the next appropriate imaging test. There are many different exams to choose from. It is often helpful to check with the radiologist. You may even get different answers from different radiologists.

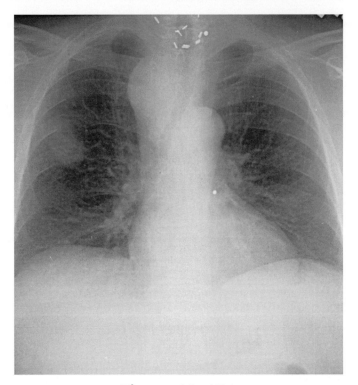

Figure 10–15A

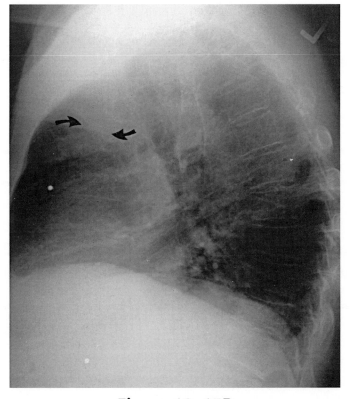

Figure 10–15B

REVIEW

I

There are _____ jokers in a deck, _____ stooges, _____ horsemen, and _____ T's in the anterior mediastinum. They are _____ , _____ , _____ , _____ , and _____ .

I _____
2/3
4/5
thyroid, thymus, teratoma, thoracic aorta, terrible lymphoma

II

For each named structure, give the mediastinal compartment:

1. esophagus _____   6. spinal nerves _____
2. heart _____   7. lymph nodes _____
3. thymus _____   8. aorta, ascending _____
4. trachea _____   9. aorta, descending _____
5. thyroid _____   10. aortic arch _____

II

1. *middle*   6. *posterior*
2. *anterior*   7. *all three*
3. *anterior*   8. *anterior*
4. *middle*   9. *middle* — ?
5. *anterior*   10. *middle*

III

In Figure 10–15*A* and *B*, the patient has multiple radiographic findings:

1. In the right lung is a (mass/nodule), located in the _____ lobe (*arrows* on lateral) in the _____ segment.
2. In addition, there is (a) [tumor/hemorrhage] in the mediastinum. Radiographic features? _____
   _____
3. The linear metallic densities at the base of the neck are surgical clips. The spherical metallic densities, however, were acquired in the cabbage patch. They are _____ . [Sign in farmer's field: "Caution, one of these cabbages has been poisoned." Sign the next morning: "Caution, two of these cabbages have been poisoned."]

   This patient had a lung cancer with metastasis to the right paratracheal nodes. The patient had a goiter removed.

III

1. *mass*
   RUL
   anterior
2. *tumor*
   It is convex, sharp, focal. It deviates, compresses, and silhouettes trachea.
   middle
3. *BB's*

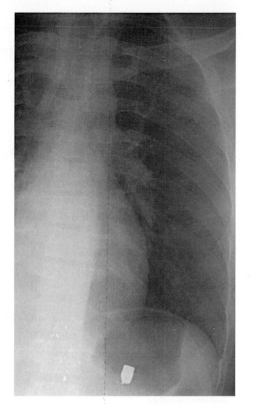

Figure 11–1A

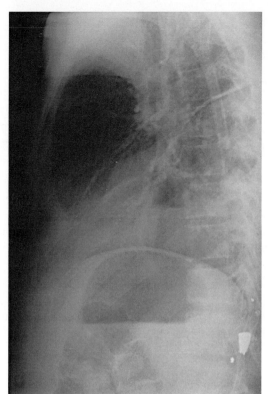

Figure 11–1B

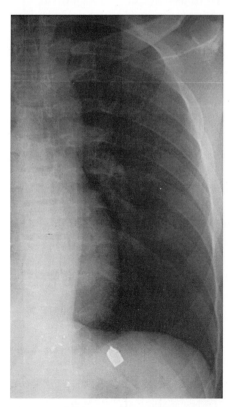

Figure 11–1C

The Pleural and Extrapleural Spaces

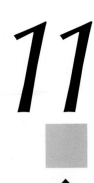

The pleural cavity is the space between the visceral and parietal pleura. The extrapleural space, a potential space, lies between the rib cage and the adherent parietal pleura. Each produces characteristic radiographic signs of disease, with the usual overlapping of signs.

1

The periphery of the base of each pleural cavity forms a rather deep gutter around the dome of the corresponding hemidiaphragm. This is called the costophrenic sulcus or angle. The deepest and most caudal portion of the _____ angle (sulcus) is posterior. The lateral costophrenic sulcus is also fairly deep.

costophrenic

2

The _____ costophrenic angle is deepest and seen only on the _____ radiograph. It is not visible on the PA radiograph because the dome of the diaphragm is [above/below] it. On the PA view, fluid is best detected in the _____ costophrenic angles.

posterior
lateral

above
lateral

3

Romeo, shown in Figure 11–1*A* and *B*, slammed the back door just as the husband fired. The bullet, almost spent, just penetrated his chest wall and dropped harmlessly into the pleural space. Figure 11–1*A* and *B* illustrates the depth of the _____ costophrenic angle as well as the hazards of sex. (Editor's note: Things were simpler in Dr. Felson's time.)

posterior

In Figure 11–1*A* (upright film), the bullet in the posterior costophrenic angle appears to lie in the abdomen. In Figure 11–1*B*, the bullet is clearly in the posterior costophrenic angle. In Figure 11–1*C* (supine film), several days later, the bullet has shifted in the pleural space.

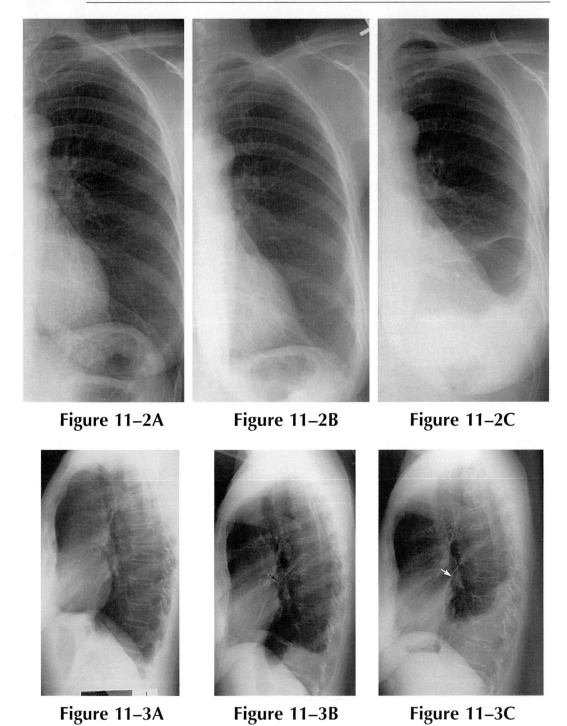

Figure 11–2A **Figure 11–2B** **Figure 11–2C**

Figure 11–3A **Figure 11–3B** **Figure 11–3C**

4

Free pleural fluid (blood, exudate, transudate, etc.) is heavier than the air-filled lung and sinks to the base of the pleural cavity in the [upright/supine] position. It causes the normally deep _____ and _____ costophrenic angles to appear shallow or blunted. In Figure 11–2A, the costophrenic sulcus is normal. In Figure 11–2B, the left costophrenic angle is _____ due to a small effusion.

5

Additional fluid will track up the pleural space, forming a meniscus, as shown in Figure 11–2C. The fluid extends higher _____ than _____ in the pleural space.

6

On the lateral x-ray, the signs are exactly the same. In Figure 11–3A, both costophrenic angles are _____ . In Figure 11–3B, the left costophrenic sulcus is _____ . In Figure 11–3C, fluid forms a _____ posteriorly. Note that the normal right costophrenic angle is visible in each.

4

upright
posterior/lateral

shallow (blunt)

5

laterally/medially

6

sharp (normal)

shallow (blunt)
meniscus

Pleural fluid is often seen tracking up the major fissure on the lateral exam, a helpful secondary sign (Fig. 11–3B and C) *(arrows)*.

Clinical Pearl: The lateral film is more sensitive than the PA film for the detection of small effusions. If there is a discrepancy between them, believe the lateral. Figures 11–2 and 11–3 are from the same patient. Compare each set of PA and lateral exams.

In Figure 11–2C, the apparent elevation of the left hemidiaphragm is actually subpulmonic fluid. The true diaphragm lies in normal position but is obscured by the parallel layer of free fluid above it. In the upright position, free fluid often collects between the lung base and the top of the diaphragm. Radiographically, the "diaphragm" appears elevated.

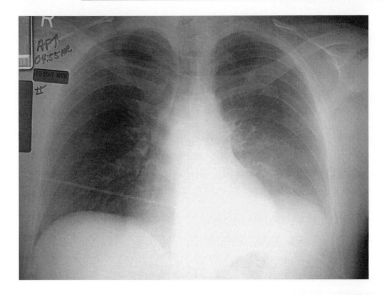

Figure 11–4A

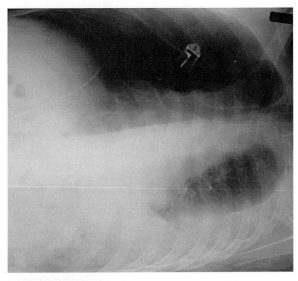

Figure 11–4B

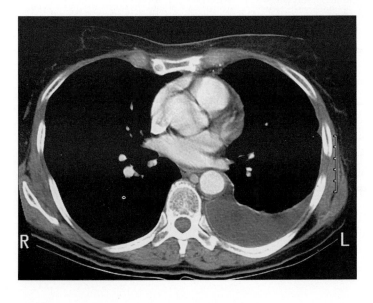

Figure 11–4C

7

As you get older, gravity is less and less a friend. In radiology, however, gravity **can be** a friend. What view would be most helpful in proving that Figure 11–4A has a subpulmonic effusion? _____ . The affected side should be [up/down] to display the layered fluid.

7

left lateral decubitus
down

Figure 11–4B is a left lateral decubitus view of the patient shown in Figure 11–4A. The free fluid has redistributed to the dependent side of the left pleural cavity, between the lung and chest wall. Figure 11–4C, a CT, demonstrates a free pleural effusion. In Figure 11–4D, ultrasound demonstrates a free effusion (E) (D = diaphragm).

8

Let's review the signs of pleural effusion on the PA radiograph. Fluid may _____ the costophrenic angle, form a _____ laterally, or hide in a _____ location. Remember, these are only seen in the [upright/supine] position.

8

blunt (fill)
meniscus
subpulmonic
upright

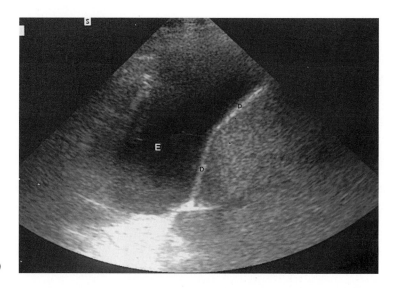

Figure 11–4D

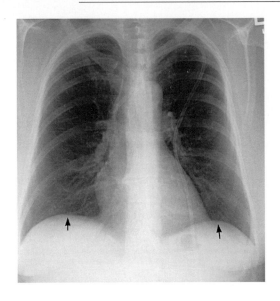

Figure 11–5A

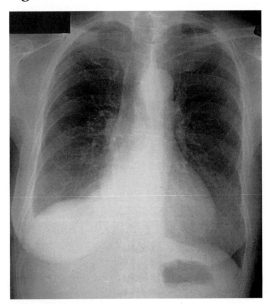

Figure 11–5B

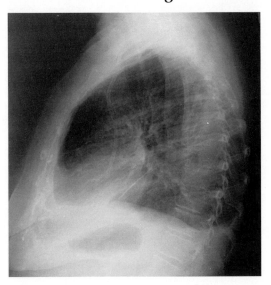

Figure 11–5C

9

We are now faced with the practical problem of recognizing subpulmonic fluid, since it so closely simulates an _____ . On the left, the stomach bubble is normally separated from the lung base by only the thin diaphragm. With left subpulmonic fluid, the gas bubble lies [farther from/closer to] the lung base. This is known as the "stomach bubble sign."

elevated hemidiaphragm

farther from

Unfortunately, there is no stomach bubble on the right. With subpulmonic effusion, often the apex of the "diaphragm" moves from a central to a lateral position, a helpful sign on either side.

Figure 11–5A is normal. The costophrenic angles are sharp, the stomach bubble is less than a centimeter from the lung, and the apex of each diaphragm *(arrow)* is in the midclavicular line.

10

What signs of effusion are seen in Figure 11–5B? Compare with Figure 11–5A.

A. On the left?

_____

B. On the right?

_____

10

A. **stomach bubble sign**

B. **diaphragmatic apex lateral, blunt costophrenic angle**

In Figure 11–5C, a lateral x-ray shows blunting of both costophrenic angles and a stomach bubble sign. There is also fluid in a major fissure.

[Handwritten notes:]

Stomach Bubble Sign

look for

Costophrenic Angle

lateral Apex

and
Stomach Bubble sign.

Also fluid in Major fissure on lat film.

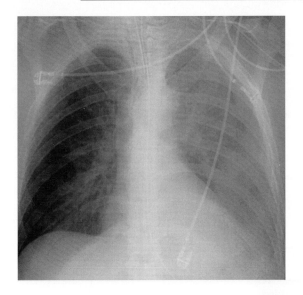

Figure 11–6

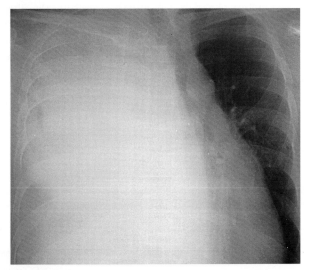

Figure 11–7A

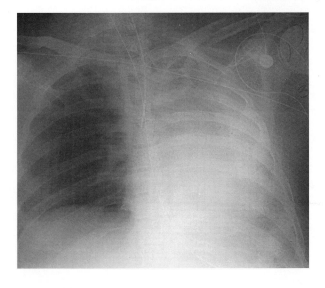

Figure 11–7B

11

With a subpulmonic effusion:

1. The "diaphragm" appears _____ .
2. The apex of the "diaphragm" may _____ .
3. The costophrenic angle may be _____ or show
   a _____ .
4. The stomach may be _____ .

11

1. *high*
2. *shift laterally*
3. *shallow (blunt)/menis-*
   cus
4. *distant from the lung*

12

In the AP supine position, the fluid gravitates [anteriorly/posteriorly] and causes the affected hemithorax to appear [more/less] radiodense. The supine patient in Figure 11–6 has a [left/right] pleural effusion. The supine view is [more/less] sensitive than the erect view in detecting effusion.

12

posteriorly
more
left
less (considerably)

Clinical Pearl: Every student wants to know how much fluid one can see on a radiograph. The erect PA requires >175 cc, the erect lateral 75 cc, the decubitus >5 cc, the supine >several hundred cc. Now you know. (Does the name Pavlov ring a bell?)

PA >175 cc
lat >75 cc
decub > 5 cc
supine > 100's

13

When one hemithorax is totally opaque, is it usually due to consolidation and atelectasis or is it due to _____ ? If the "white lung" is due to atelectasis, the mediastinum shifts [toward/away from] the lesion. If the "white lung" is due to pleural fluid, it shifts [toward/away from] the lesion.

13

pleural effusion
toward

away from

14

Compare the "white lungs" of Figure 11–7A and B.
A. Figure 11–7A is due to _____ .
   Why? _____ .
B. Figure 11–7B is due to _____ .
   Why? _____ .

14

A. *pleural effusion*
   contralateral shift
B. *atelectasis*
   ipsilateral shift

Clinical Pearl: If there is a "white hemithorax" but *no shift,* both atelectasis and effusion may be present. There is a balance between collapse and pleural fluid. This is most often due to lung cancer.

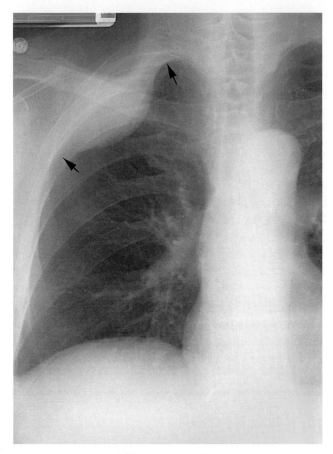

Figure 11–8A

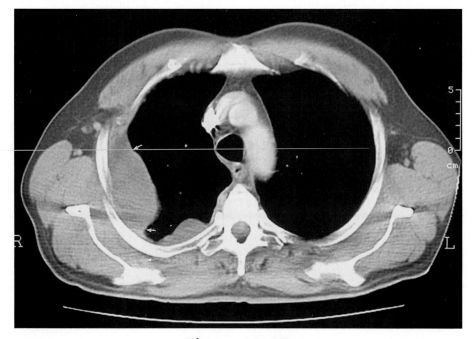

Figure 11–8B

15

Encapsulated (loculated) pleural effusion is attributable to pleural adhesions, preexisting or developing after the appearance of the fluid. It [does/does not] shift within changing positions.

15

does not

16

Loculated fluid may simulate lung disease. Consult Figure 11–8A, an example of loculated pleural fluid. The borders of an encapsulation are generally [concave/convex] toward the lung. The margin forms an [obtuse/acute] angle with the chest wall when seen in profile *(arrows)*. An air bronchogram is [present/absent].

16

convex

obtuse

absent

Figure 11–8B, a CT of the loculated fluid, shows a similar appearance. Compare this with the free effusion of Figure 11–4C (p. 184).

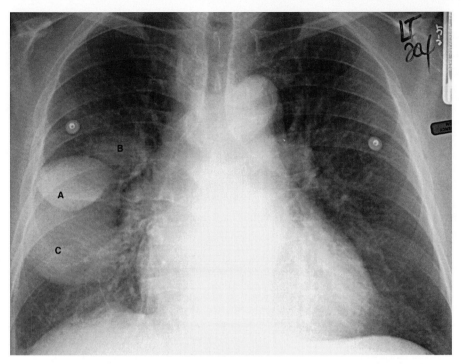

Figure 11–9A

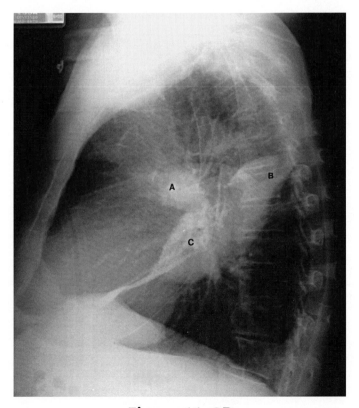

Figure 11–9B

17

Occasionally, a focal *intrafissural* fluid collection may look like a lung mass. Because it splits the fissure, this "pseudotumor" is often [lenticular/spherical] in shape.

18

Intrafissural effusion ("pseudotumor") is bounded by visceral pleura and its margins appear [sharp/hazy] when seen in profile (on edge). The encapsulated effusion in the *minor fissure* should have sharp margins in [PA/LAT/both] view(s). The margins of the "mass" in the *major fissure* should be sharp in the [PA/lateral/both] view(s). (Remember, the beam must be parallel to the fissure to see it.)

17

lenticular

18

sharp

both

lateral

Figure 11–9*A* and *B* shows that the minor fissure "pseudotumor" (A) has sharp margins in the PA and lateral. The two loculated collections in the major fissure (B and C) are sharp only in the lateral projection. Note the tapering edges (lens shape).

Clinical Pearl: "Pseudotumors" are most commonly encountered in congestive heart failure. As the CHF resolves, the loculated fluid disappears ("vanishing tumor").

Intrafissural
Effusion
↓
Pseudotumor

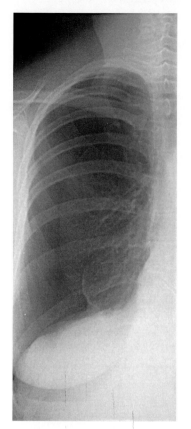

Figure 11–10A

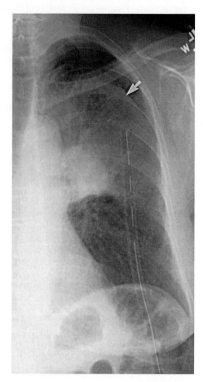

Figure 11–10B

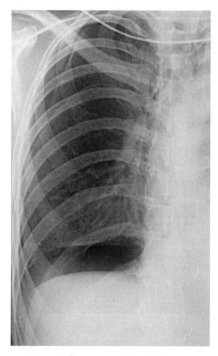

Figure 11–11

19

Air in the pleural space is [more/less] radiolucent than the lung. With a pneumothorax, the visceral pleura is seen as a thin white line between air in the _____ and air in the _____ . When the lung is consolidated, the pneumothorax appears as an _____ adjacent to the air in the pleural space.

19

more

lung
pleural space
edge

Figure 11–10*A* shows the pleura on end between the pleural air and the aerated lung. Figure 11–10*B* shows the pleural air against the edge of the consolidated upper lobe *(arrow).*

20

In the supine patient, air collects anteriorly, laterally, and _____ . In Figure 11–11, we see what two signs of pneumothorax? _____ and _____ . Note the subpulmonic air.

20

inferiorly
hyperlucent pleural space
visceral pleural line

21

The supine film is [more/less] sensitive than the erect film for detecting pneumothorax. If the patient cannot sit or stand, the _____ position may be substituted. The side in question should be _____ .

21

less

decubitus
up

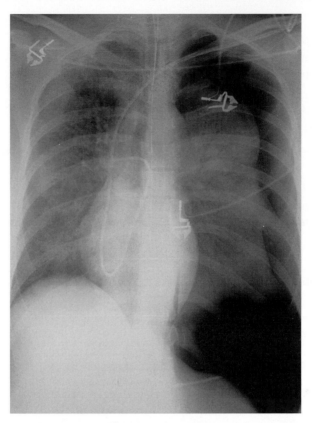

Figure 11–12

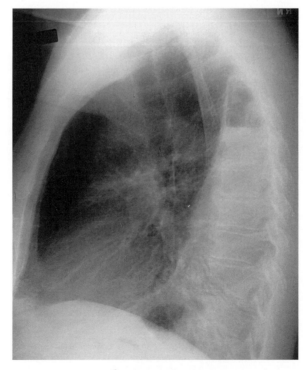

Figure 11–13

22

Occasionally, air enters the pleural space with each breath but cannot escape, increasing the intrapleural pressure. The pressure change (elevates/depresses) the diaphragm, collapses the lung, and shifts the mediastinum (toward/away from) the pneumothorax. This is known as a "tension pneumothorax."

22

depresses (flattens)

away from

23

Tension pneumothorax compromises pulmonary venous return and is a medical emergency. The three radiographic signs are _____ , _____ , and _____ .

23

depressed diaphragm/ shifted mediastinum/collapsed lung

Figure 11–12 shows a tension pneumothorax with collapsed lung, a depressed diaphragm, and a mediastinal shift to the right.

Clinical Pearl: Rapid decompression of a tension pneumothorax can be lifesaving. Learn the clinical signs so you can diagnose and treat it without an x-ray. Signs include rapid onset of respiratory failure, decreased breath sounds, deviated trachea, and jugular venous distention.

24

A hydropneumothorax is air and fluid in the pleural space. On the erect film, the lower pleural space will appear _____ , the upper pleural space will appear _____ , and a(n) _____ will be visible at their interface.

24

radiodense
radiolucent
air/fluid level

Figure 11–13 shows fluid in the lower pleural space, air in the upper pleural space, and an air/fluid level.

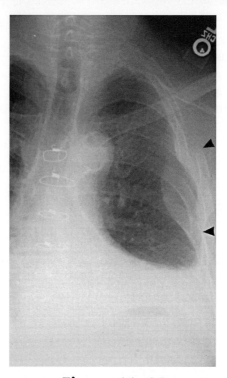

Figure 11–14

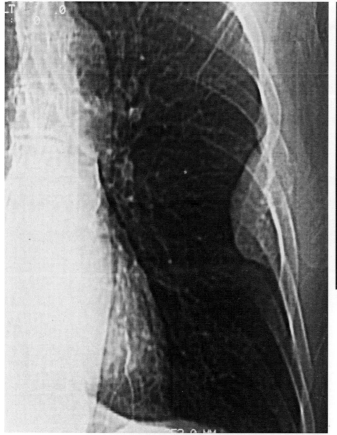

Figure 11–15A

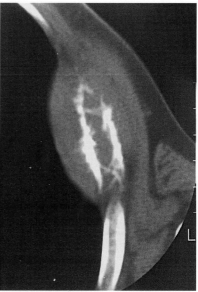

Figure 11–15B

25

The extrapleural space is a potential space that lies between the rib cage and the _____ . Lesions that arise in structures within or bordering the extrapleural space (ribs, muscle, connective tissue, etc.) may lift the adjacent parietal pleura and push it toward the _____ . A typical extrapleural lesion is convex with a [sharp/hazy] interface with the lung. It forms an [acute/obtuse] angle with the chest wall when viewed in tangent.

26

A focal intrapleural lesion (encapsulated fluid) and an extrapleural lesion can both form [acute/obtuse] angles with the chest wall and a [sharp/hazy] lung interface. The presence of a rib lesion indicates a [pleural/extrapleural] origin. If none is visible, it may be difficult to separate the two.

25

parietal pleura

lung
sharp
obtuse

26

obtuse
sharp
extrapleural

Figure 11–14 illustrates an extrapleural hematoma. The convex margin facing the lung is *sharp* and the borders are *tapered* (obtuse angle with chest wall). It looks very similar to encapsulated fluid (Fig. 11–8A, p. 190). The rib fractures *(arrowheads)* indicate the extrapleural origin.

27

Cross-sectional imaging helps separate extrapleural from intrapleural lesions by eliminating overlap of structures. Figure 11–15A, a computed radiograph, shows a mass that forms an [acute/obtuse] angle with the chest wall. The CT in Figure 11–15B shows that this mass is [intra/extra] pleural. Why? _____

27

obtuse
extra
expansile rib lesion, soft tissue mass

Clinical Pearl: Most extrapleural lesions are due to rib fractures and rib metastasis.

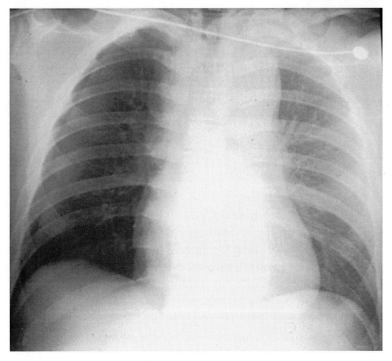

Figure 11–16A

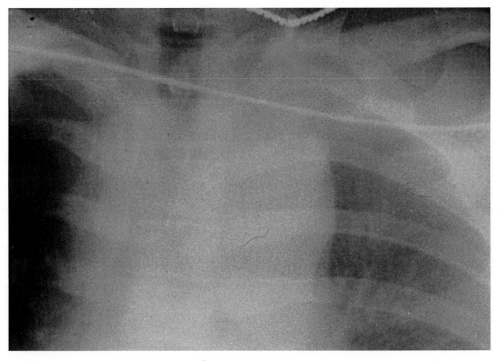

Figure 11–16B

REVIEW

I

A. What are the three patterns with *free* pleural effusions seen on an erect film?
1. _Blont costophrenic Angle_
2. _Meniscus_
3. _Subpulmonic effusion_

B. List four clues to a subpulmonic effusion:
1. _Diaphragm appears high_
2. _Stomach Bubble sign_
3. _Diaphram Apex is late_
4. _see A: 1,2_

A,B: may see from 2N fissure.

II

To diagnose a pneumothorax, one must see:
1. _____
2. _____

III

Figure 11–16 is a supine x-ray of a young woman who was in an auto accident.

A. On the left, there is [increased/decreased] radiodensity, most likely due to _____ .

B. On the right, there is [increased/decreased] radiolucency laterally, due to _____ .

C. The mediastinum is [normal/focally widened/generally widened], most likely due to _____ .

I

A. 1. **blunt costophrenic angle**
2. **meniscus**
3. **subpulmonic effusion**

B. 1. **high "diaphragm"**
2. **stomach bubble sign**
3. **"diaphragm" apex is lateral**
4. **shallow costophrenic angles/thickened fissure**

II

1. **peripheral hyperlucency (intrapleural air)**
2. **visceral pleural line or edge**

III

A. **increased/layered pleural fluid (blood)**
B. **increased/ pneumothorax**
C. **generally widened/ hemorrhage**

"In the field of observation, chance favors the prepared mind."—Louis Pasteur

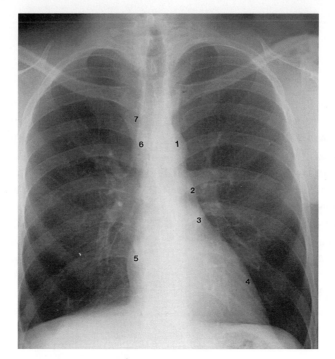

Figure 12–1A

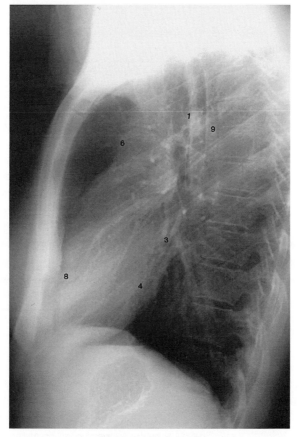

Figure 12–1B

Cardiovascular Disease

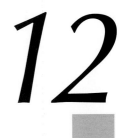

12

The heart is an anterior mediastinal structure. To analyze cardiovascular disease fully, however, the heart, pulmonary vessels, lungs, and pleural space must all be studied. Every beginner should be able to recognize the cardiovascular structures, cardiomegaly, and left heart failure. If *you* can, you will be ahead of most of your peers. (Two medical students spotted a bear while walking in the woods. Student #1 took out sneakers from his backpack and put them on. "You can't outrun a bear," said Student #2. Said Student #1, "I don't have to, I just have to outrun you.")

1

Figure 12–1*A* is a diagram of the heart and great vessels. On the left side, there are four bulges (moguls to you skiers). They are:

1. _____   3. _____
2. _____   4. _____

Note: The *normal* left atrial appendage is concave, not convex.

1

1. aortic arch
2. main pulmonary artery
3. left atrial appendage
4. left ventricle

2

The right heart border is formed by the _____ (5). The right ventricle does not form a lateral border on the frontal view. Above the right heart border is the _____ (6). The _____ (7) is parallel to the upper mediastinum.

2

5. right atrium
6. ascending aorta
7. superior vena cava

3

On the lateral film, the right heart is anterior and the left heart is posterior. Label the cardiovascular structures on the lateral (Figure 12–1*B*).

1 _____   6 _____
3 _____   8 _____
4 _____   9 _____

3

1. aortic arch
3. left atrium
4. left ventricle
6. ascending aorta
8. right ventricle
9. descending aorta
   (proximal)

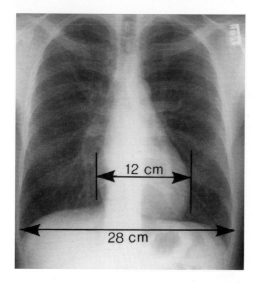

Figure 12–2

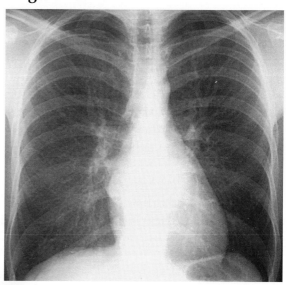

Figure 12–3A

left Atrial
Enlargement
(Normal Pm "Concave")

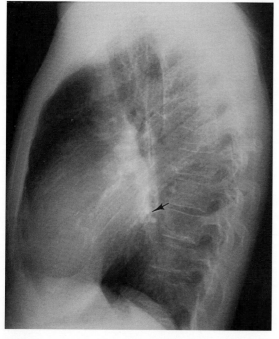

Figure 12–3B

4

Sometimes the terminology is confusing. Review the following:

A. The left heart sits [anterior/posterior] to the right heart.
B. On the frontal view, the right heart border is the _____ only.
C. On the frontal view, the left atrial appendage is normally [concave/convex].

4

A. posterior
B. right atrium
C. concave

Determining cardiac enlargement is easy. Measure the horizontal width of the heart and divide it by the widest internal diameter of the thorax. The normal cardiothoracic ratio is less than 0.5 (oversimplified, but useful).

5

In Figure 12–2, the cardiothoracic ratio is _____ .
The upper limit of normal is _____ .

5

0.43 (12/28)
0.50

Clinical Pearl: The cardiothoracic ratio is based on population standards. For a given patient, an increase of greater than 1 cm in cardiac diameter from a prior film is a more reliable index of cardiac enlargement than the cardiothoracic ratio. In general, a radiologist with a ruler is a radiologist in trouble, but these measurements work fairly well on erect, inspiratory PA radiographs.

6

The "heart" may be enlarged due to intrinsic cardiac disease or surrounding pericardial fluid. Unfortunately, the x-ray does not distinguish between cardiac _____ and pericardial _____ . Many prefer the term "cardiac silhouette" to "heart size" for this reason.

6

enlargement
fluid

7

If the left atrium enlarges, it protrudes [laterally/medially] and [anteriorly/posteriorly]. On the frontal view, its margin becomes [concave/convex].

7

laterally
posteriorly
convex

Figure 12–3A and B show an enlarged left atrium. The upper left heart border bulges laterally and posteriorly *(arrow)*. Compare with Figure 12–1A and B.

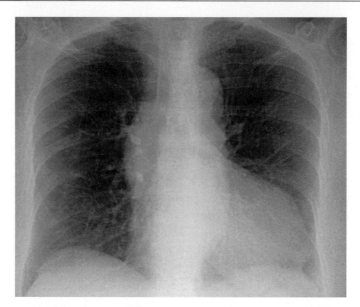

Figure 12–4A

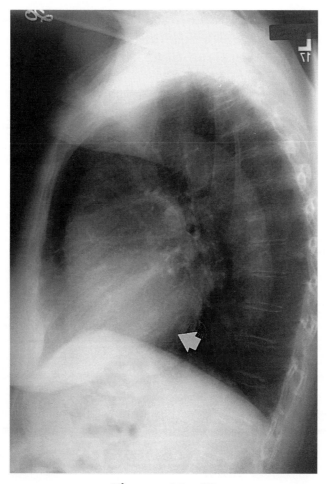

Figure 12–4B

8

If the left ventricle enlarges on the PA film, the lower left heart border moves [laterally/medially] and the cardiac apex moves inferiorly. On the lateral film, it protrudes [anteriorly/posteriorly] and inferiorly.

8

laterally

posteriorly

Figure 12–4*A* and *B* shows left ventricular enlargement. On the frontal view, the heart border moves laterally, and the cardiac apex moves inferolaterally. On the lateral view, the left heart border moves inferoposteriorly *(arrow)*. Compare with Figure 12–3*A* and *B*. Also note the tortuous aorta on the PA and lateral.

9

To review: A large left atrium will bulge _____ on the PA film and _____ on the lateral film. A large left ventricle will bulge _____ on the PA film and _____ on the lateral film.

9

laterally
posteriorly
laterally and inferiorly
posteriorly and inferiorly

left heart
Enlargement

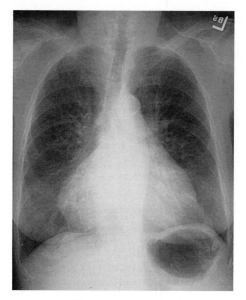

Figure 12–5A

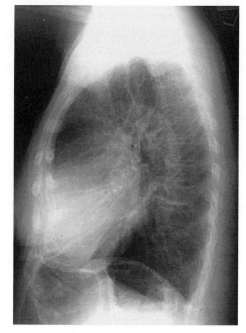

Figure 12–5B

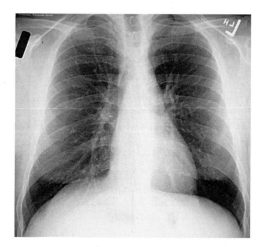

Figure 12–6

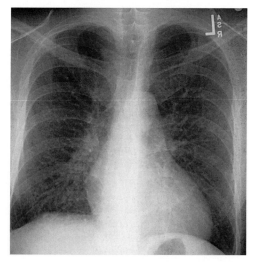

Figure 12–7

Detecting right heart enlargement is more difficult. In the frontal projection, the normal right heart protrudes slightly to the right of the spine and an enlarged right heart protrudes further to the right (soft science, at best). In the lateral projection, the right heart enlarges anteriorly and superiorly. The normal right heart contacts the lower one-third of the sternum, while the enlarged heart contacts the lower one-half. Compare the enlarged right heart (Fig. 12–5) with the enlarged left heart in Figure 12–4.

RT heart

10

Many heart diseases also alter the pulmonary vessels. In a normal erect patient, gravity causes the majority of blood to flow to the [apex/base]. In Figure 12–6, the upper lobe vessels are [larger/smaller] than the lower lobe vessels at approximately the same distance from the hilum. In a supine patient, what happens to blood flow?

_____

10

base
smaller

Apical
apex = base

11

In Figure 12–7, the upper lobe vessels are [larger/smaller] than the lower lobe vessels. This is called cephalization or vascular redistribution. Cephalization, not heart size, is the key to diagnosing elevated left heart pressure. Compare Figure 12–7 and Figure 12–6 until cephalization is absolutely clear.

11
larger

Cephalization or Vascular Redistribution

Clinical Pearl: Left heart failure and mitral valve stenosis are the most frequent causes of redistribution or cephalization.

The patient in Figure 12–7 is in left heart failure. The cardiothoracic ratio is over 0.5 and there is cephalization of the upper lobe vessels. This is mild left heart failure because the vessel margins remain distinct (i.e., no edema).

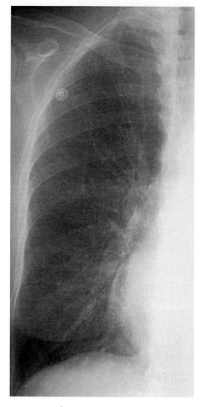

Figure 12–8A

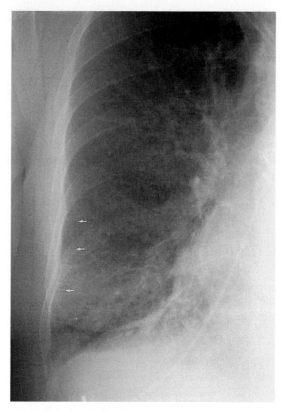

Figure 12–8B

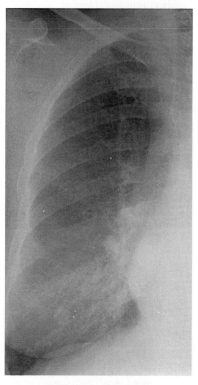

Figure 12–8C

12

As the left atrial pressure increases, interstitial edema de-velops. The edema causes the vessel margins to be-come _____ and the peripheral interstitial mark-ings to become _____ .

12

indistinct (unsharp)
prominent

Figure 12–8*A* shows mild left heart failure. The upper and lower lobe vessels are equal and there is no edema. Figure 12–8*B* shows moderate heart failure with large but indistinct upper lobe vessels and prominent interstitium. Fluid may thicken the interlobular septa, causing short lines perpendicular to the pleural surface. These are "Kerley B" lines indicating interstitial edema *(arrows).*

Kerley B

13

In Figure 12–8*A*, the costophrenic angle is _____ .
In Figure 12–8*B*, the costophrenic sulcus is _____ ,
indicating _____ . Pleural effusion is frequent in moderate to severe CHF.

13

sharp
shallow (blunt)
pleural fluid (effusion)

14

In Figure 12–8*C*, there is evidence of severe edema. The edema tends to be more severe in the gravity-dependent [upper/lower] lungs. With alveolar edema, the pulmonary vessels may not be visible. Why? _____

14

lower
water density lung around
water density vessels

Figure 12–8*A–C* are from the same patient. Study the progression from cephaliza-tion to interstitial edema to alveolar edema.

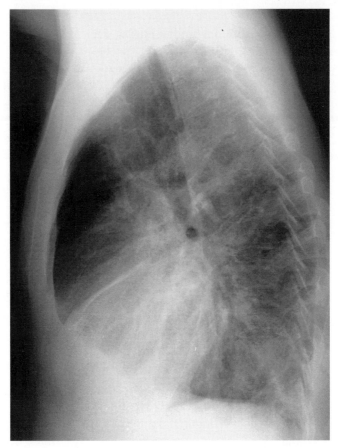

Figure 12–9

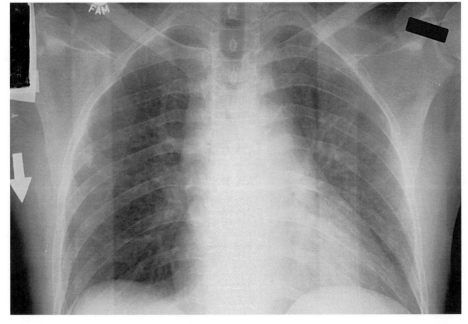

Figure 12–10

15

In left heart failure, the cardiac silhouette often enlarges. In addition:

1. In mild failure, there is ~~cephalization~~ of the vessels, but no edema.
2. Moderate failure causes indistinct vessel margins, ~~interstitial~~ edema, and ~~Kerley~~ lines. Pleural effusions may be present.
3. Severe failure causes ~~Alveolar~~ edema and pleural effusions.

15

~~✗~~

1. *cephalization*

2. *interstitial/Kerley*

3. *alveolar*

16

On the lateral radiograph, Figure 12–9, describe three findings that confirm the congestive heart failure.

1 _____ 3 _____

2 _____

16

1. *pleural effusion (thick fissure)*
2. *edema*
3. *big left ventricle/vascular redistribution*

Clinical Pearl: With cephalization, lung auscultation is usually normal. With interstitial edema, crackling rales are audible. With alveolar edema, rales (wet crackles) are audible.

17

Figure 12–10 is a portable radiograph.

1. It is taken [supine/erect].
2. The cardiothoracic ratio is _____ (AP FILM)
3. The upper lobe pulmonary vessels are _____ .
4. Patient [is/is not/can't tell] in heart failure.

? May have effusion.

17

1. *supine (down arrow)*
2. *not valid*
3. *normal for supine*
4. *can't tell*

Tend to lower when supine.

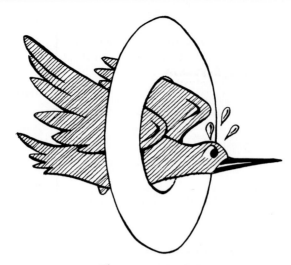

Figure 12–11

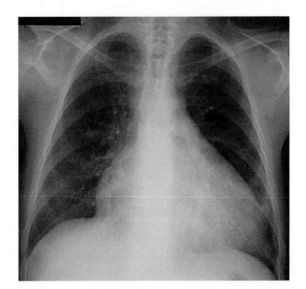

Figure 12–12

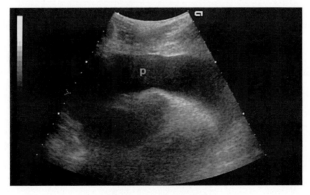

Figure 12–13

18

Name the physiologist whose law described the relationship between edema, hydrostatic pressure, and oncotic pressure: _____ . Figure 12–11 is a _____ .

18

Starling
Starling resistor

19

In Figure 12–12, cardiac silhouette is enlarged. Is there cephalization? _____ . Is there edema? _____ Is there pleural effusion? _____ . There are no significant signs of left heart failure. Perhaps the large cardiac silhouette is due to a _____ .

19

no
no/no

pericardial effusion

In Figure 12–13, an echocardiogram shows a large pericardial effusion (P). In Figure 12–14, a CT shows a pericardial effusion (P), bilateral pleural effusions, and LUL consolidation. Echocardiography, CT, and MRI accurately depict pericardial effusions, but echocardiology is most cost effective.

Clinical Pearl: Marked enlargement of the cardiac silhouette, with no or mild signs of left heart failure, is most likely due to pericardial effusion. Cardiomyopathy and multivalvular heart disease may have a similar radiographic presentation.

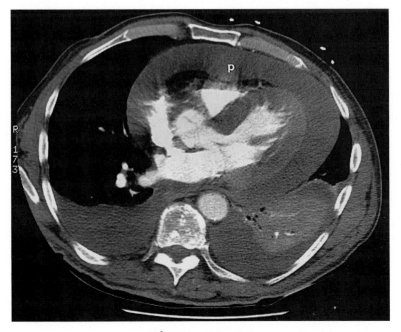

Figure 12–14

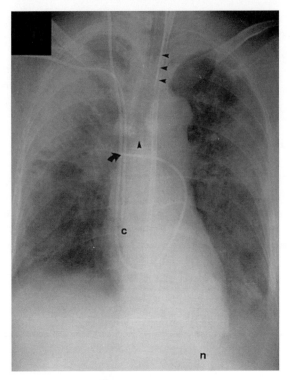

Figure 12–15

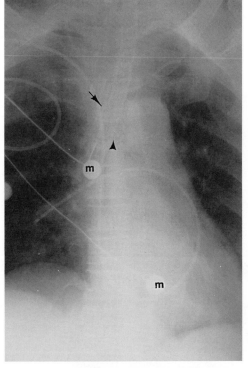

Figure 12–16

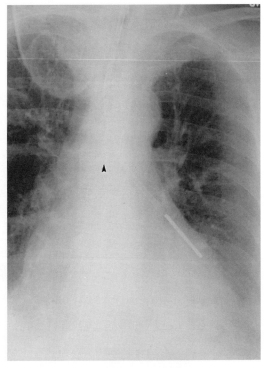

Figure 12–17

BONUS SECTION

Patients with heart or lung disease often wind up in the ICU with many support tubes and catheters. These should be evaluated on every x-ray before you start your standard search.

20

In Figure 12–15, the apparatus is correctly positioned:
A. Endotracheal tube (arrowheads) with its tip [at the carina/in the midtrachea/in the cervical trachea].
B. Central venous catheter (c) in the _____ .
C. Nasogastric tube tip (n) in the _____ .
D. The Swan-Ganz catheter tip (arrow) is in the _____ . (vertical arrowhead = carina)

20

A. *in the midtrachea*
B. *superior vena cava or proximal right atrium*
C. *stomach*
D. *right main pulmonary artery*

21

In Figure 12–16, extraneous wires overlie the chest. The monitoring electrodes (m) are external. Now troubleshoot the rest.
A. The endotracheal tube is in the _____ .
B. The CPV catheter tip (arrow) is in the _____ .
C. The Swan-Ganz catheter tip is in the _____ .

21

A. *right main stem bronchus*
B. *superior vena cava*
C. *right lower lobe artery (too peripheral)*

22

In Figure 11–7B (p. 188), why is the left lung collapsed? _____ .

22

endotracheal tube, right main bronchus

23

Figure 12–17. History. "Patient with tracheostomy. Check feeding tube position." The feeding tube is in the _____ .

23

left lower lobe bronchus

Congratulations! You are done. ("He who laughs, lasts." Leo Rosten)

There will be no review quiz. Take a break! When you come back, challenge yourself to the great quiz cases in the last section. Also be sure to read the "Ten Axioms for a Lifetime of Learning in Medicine."

Felson's 10 Axioms for a Lifetime of Learning Medicine

1. If you like it, you'll learn it; so learn to like it.

2. Principles are as important as facts. If you master the principles, you can make up the facts.

3. You learn better when you know your goals. If you don't now where you're going, says the Talmud, all roads will take you there. But if you do know, you'll get there much quicker.

4. Follow your cases. I've learned and remembered more by followup than any other way. It's hard work, but as Confucius say, "He learneth most who worketh most." Or was it Knute Rockne?

5. Like sex, learning is better if you are actively involved. When you read, talk back to the author. Be skeptical. Don't follow the authorities too closely or you may become a Brown Nose Duck; he can fly as fast as the leader, but can't stop as quick.

6. Reinforcement is essential for acquiring knowledge. But don't reinforce by simple repetition; use some other method than the original way you learned it. See a case, look it up; read an article, find a case or ask a question.

7. Reward is important for learning. Show off what you know. Brag a little. Speak up in class. Tell your spouse or sweetheart; tell your colleagues; don't bother to tell your friends—you won't have any.

8. Different people learn best by different methods. Figure out your own best method and cater to it, whether it be reading, listening, observing, or doing, or a combination of these. Don't depend on great teachers. They are as rare as great students.

9. Quick retrieval of once-acquired information is crucial. The home computer is ideal but other good retrieval methods are available. Create your own personal modification and keep improving it. Without a recall system you're a "loser," an old man with a stuck zipper.

10. Divide your study time into prime time, work time, and sleepy time. Biorhythms vary widely among students, so develop your own study schedule. Don't watch television during prime time and don't read medicine during sleepy time.

Felson, B. *Humor in Medicine,* 1989; RHA Inc., Cincinnati, Ohio.

Quiz
"Ten Great Cases"

CHALLENGE: Each case tests your ability to apply the fundamental principles we have just gone over and over and over.

SUGGESTIONS:
1. Read the history.
2. Evaluate the x-ray with your routine scanning pattern (ATMLL), making all the pertinent observations.
3. Then, and only then, answer *all* questions before you turn to the answers on the next page.

Beware of *"satisfaction of search."* There is a tendency when reading x-rays to be so thrilled that you have actually found an abnormality that you then relax your search. Don't! Many patients have several abnormalities that you can combine to arrive at a diagnosis.

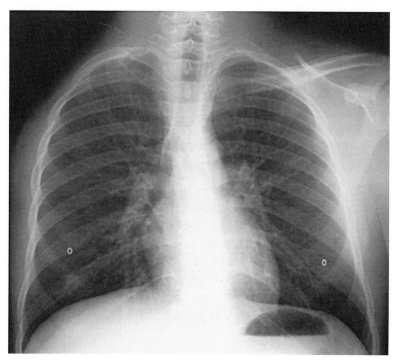

Figure Q–1

CASE 1 _____

HISTORY: Young Male With Cancer.

Metal nipple markers have been placed to distinguish nipples, which sometimes show on x-rays, from real pulmonary nodules.

1. Is the lung abnormal? _____ If so, where? _____ What? _____

2. Are there any changes to suggest pleural effusion? _____ If so, what? _____

3. What type of surgery did the patient have? _____

4. Can you combine the history and x-ray findings in 1 and 3 to suggest a diagnosis? _____

■◆■ CASE 1

1. Yes, below the right nipple marker, where the ribs cross, there is a pulmonary nodule.
2. No. The costophrenic angles are sharp. The stomach bubble sign is absent. Diaphragms are normally shaped.
3. The right shoulder has been amputated. A systematic approach helps save embarrassing misses.
4. Patient had a shoulder amputation for osteosarcoma. The nodule is a pulmonary metastasis, a frequent occurrence in all sarcomas.

"Intuition is the source of scientific knowledge." Aristotle
"Aristotle could have avoided the mistake of thinking that women have fewer teeth than men by the simple device of asking Mrs. Aristotle to open her mouth." Bertrand Russell

■◆■

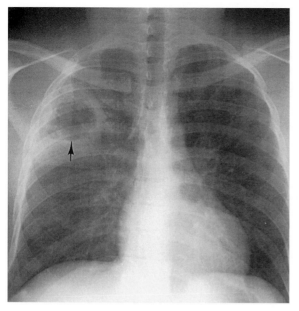

Figure Q–2A

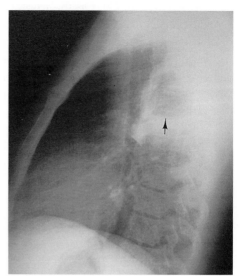

Figure Q–2B

■◆■ CASE 2

HISTORY: This Is A 30-Year-Old Epileptic With High Fever And Chills For 5 Days.

1. The obvious abnormality is [pleural/parenchymal/extrapleural/can't tell].

2. Describe the lesion in detail _____.

3. The arrow points to a/an _____.

4. In what lobe is it located? _____ What segment? _____

5. Put the x-ray findings and history together for a logical diagnosis.

■◆■ CASE 2

1. It is parenchymal. On the frontal, it may be difficult to tell, but on the lateral, it sits just anterior to the major fissure, clearly within the lung.
2. There is a mass or focal alveolar consolidation with a central cavity.
3. The arrow points to an air/fluid level.
4. Right upper lobe, posterior segment—it sits on the major fissure.
5. This is a lung abscess in an epileptic who probably aspirated during a seizure. Tuberculosis, another reasonable thought, is usually more indolent. Aspiration most often involves the posterior segment of the upper lobe and the superior and posterior basal segments of the lower lobe. These segments are gravity dependent in the supine patient.

"It's what you learn after you know it all that counts." Earl Weaver

■◆■

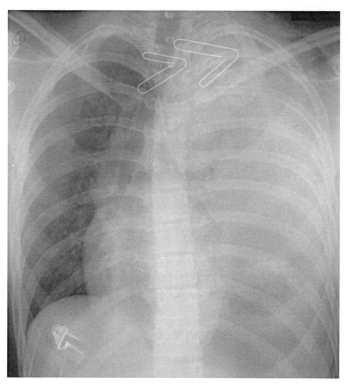

Figure Q–3

■◆■ CASE 3 _____

HISTORY: This Hypotensive Patient Has A Gunshot Wound To The Left Chest.

Identical paper clips mark the entrance and exit wounds.

1. This radiograph is most likely [erect/supine] (PA/AP).

2. Describe the major radiologic findings on the left. _____
   What is the most likely cause? _____

3. Are proximal air bronchograms visible? _____ What does this tell
   you? _____

4. The police tell us he was shot from the front. Is the entry wound midline or left-
   sided? _____
   How did you decide? _____

■◆■ CASE 3

1. Supine, AP—patient is hypotensive.
2. The left hemithorax is opaque and the mediastinum is shifted to the contralateral side. There is a large left pleural effusion, undoubtedly blood. There is also some subcutaneous air over the left shoulder.
3. Yes, the air bronchogram on the left tells us that the major airways are open. There is no central endobronchial obstruction and the surrounding lung is airless (water density).
4. Left-sided. This is an AP supine film; therefore the anterior clip will be magnified. Since identical paper clips were used, the bullet must have entered the left chest and exited in the midline.

"Why shouldn't truth be stranger than fiction? Fiction has to be believable." Mark Twain

■◆■

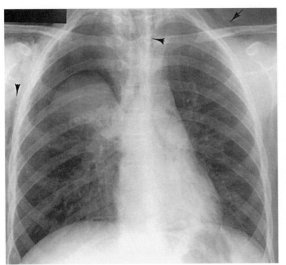

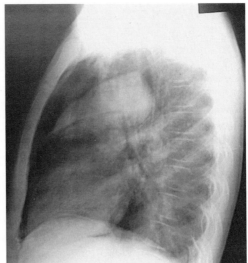

Figure Q–4A   **Figure Q–4B**

■◆■ **CASE 4** _____

HISTORY: 11-Year-Old Child With Asthma And Fever For Two Days. Then He Suddenly Became Short Of Breath.

1. There is consolidation of the _____ lobe.

2. The lucency above the consolidated lobe is due to _____.

3. The linear black streaks *(arrows)* over the mediastinum, chest wall, and base of the neck are due to _____.

4. Combine history and x-ray finding to formulate a diagnosis. _____

■◆■ CASE 4

1. Right upper lobe.
2. Pneumothorax (see edge of consolidated lung).
3. Pneumomediastinum and subcutaneous emphysema of the chest wall and neck.
4. This is an asthmatic who developed a pneumonia. The pneumothorax, pneumomediastinum, and subcutaneous emphysema are due to barotrauma from a combination of air trapping due to bronchospasm and vigorous coughing.

"He's crazy; he thinks he's a chicken." "Why don't you take him to a psychiatrist?" "I can't, we need the eggs." Woody Allen
"Schizophrenia beats dining alone." Oscar Lavant

■◆■

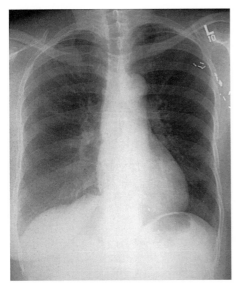

Figure Q–5A

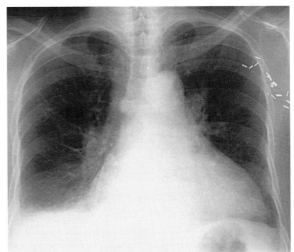

Figure Q–5B

■◆■ CASE 5

HISTORY: This Is A 50-Year-Old Woman. In Figure Q–5A, She Was Asymptomatic. In Figure Q–5B, 10 Months Later, She Has Pain On Inspiration.

1. In Figure Q–5A, are the two lungs equally radiolucent? _____ Explain the discrepancy. _____

2. Ten months later, there have been two striking changes.
   A. Figure Q–5B. The cardiac size (cardiac silhouette) is _____, while the pulmonary vessels are unchanged. This suggests what diagnosis? _____
   B. Figure Q–5B. The patient has a new [right/left] [pleural effusion/pneumothorax]. Radiographic findings? _____

3. Combining the history and your radiographic observations, the most likely diagnosis is _____ and _____ caused by _____.

■◆■ CASE 5

1. The left lung is more lucent. There has been a left mastectomy. The breast is missing and there are clips in the axilla. There is less soft tissue on the left, so there is less absorption of radiation.
2. A. Enlarged. Pericardial effusion.
   B. Right pleural effusion. The right costophrenic angle is blunt and there is a small meniscus. The right diaphragm has also changed shape (subpulmonic effusion).
3. Pericardial effusion *and* right pleural effusion *caused by* metastatic breast cancer.

"I like only two kinds of men: domestic and imported." Mae West
"She may be good for nothing, but she's not bad for nothing." Mae West

■◆■

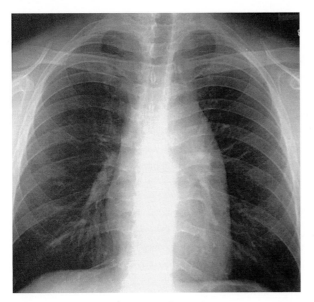

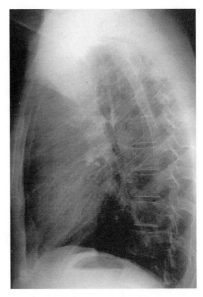

Figure Q–6A   **Figure Q–6B**

■◆■ CASE 6

HISTORY: Young Male Without Symptoms.

1. There is a large intrathoracic mass. It causes a silhouette sign of what three cardiovascular structures? _____, _____, and _____

2. Where is this mass seen on the lateral film? _____

3. In which mediastinal compartment(s) is this mass? _____

4. Present a differential diagnosis. _____

■◆■ CASE 6

1. The left atrium, pulmonary artery, and the aortic arch (knob).
2. Retrosternal clear space, between sternum and trachea.
3. This is a large anterior and middle mediastinal mass on the left. The lateral radiograph shows the mass in the anterior mediastinum. The silhouette sign indicates anterior mediastinum (left atrium) and middle mediastinum (pulmonary artery, aortic knob).
4. Remember the "5 T's." The mass is too low for thyroid. The ascending thoracic aorta is on the right. Terrible lymphoma is usually lobulated. Thymoma and teratoma are the best choices. (It is not uncommon for large masses to cross mediastinal boundaries.)

"If law school is so hard to get through, how come there are so many lawyers?" Calvin Trillin

"Health food makes me sick." Calvin Trillin

■◆■

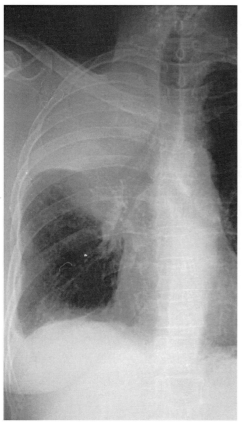

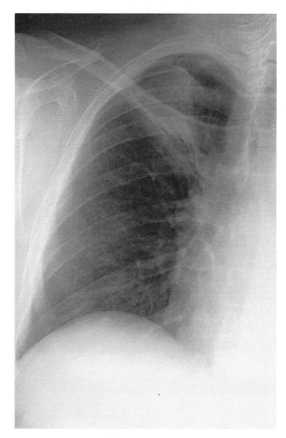

Figure Q–7A   **Figure Q–7B**

■◆■ CASE 7

HISTORY: These Are Two Older Women, Both With A Cough.

1. What lobe is involved? _____

2. What forms the sharp lower edges of their lesions? _____ Reason?
_____

3. A. Patient [A/B] has consolidation due to a central obstruction. Radiographic findings: _____
   B. Patient [A/B] has peripheral ~~resorptive~~ *obstructive* atelectasis. Radiographic findings: _____ *P5 125.*

4. Patient [A/B] probably has lung cancer. Patient [A/B] probably has a community acquired pneumonia.

■◆■ CASE 7

1. Right upper lobe.
2. The minor fissure is the sharp lower border. The upper lobe is consolidated (airspace or alveolar disease) and the middle lobe is well aerated.
3. A. Patient A has postobstructive atelectasis and consolidation. There is no air bronchogram and little volume loss. Patient A also has a right pleural effusion (blunt costophrenic sulcus) and a right hilar mass (compare with patient B).
   B. Patient B has atelectasis but open airways. The minor fissure is elevated and there is an air bronchogram partially hidden behind the clavicle.
4. **Diagnosis:** Patient A has a carcinoma obstructing the right upper lobe bronchus (i.e., no right upper lobe air bronchogram). Patient B has alveolar infiltrate or air space consolidation due to a community-acquired pneumonia.

"An onion can make people cry but there's never been a vegetable that can make people laugh." Will Rogers
"We are all here for a spell, get all the good laughs you can." Will Rogers

■◆■

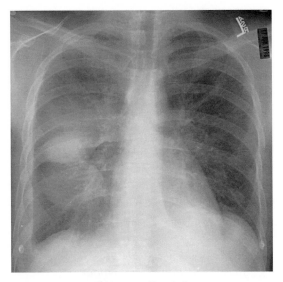

Figure Q–8A

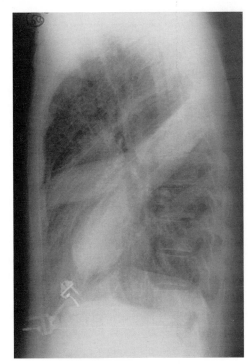

Figure Q–8B

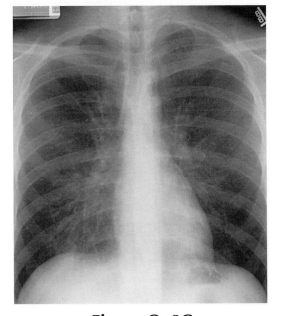

Figure Q–8C

■◆■ CASE 8 ───

HISTORY: This is a 60-year-old patient with increasing shortness of breath over several days (Figs. Q–8A and 8B). Fortunately, his x-ray jacket contains a film done 6 months earlier (Fig. Q–8C).

1. What has happened to the heart size in the interval? _____
2. What has happened to the pulmonary vessels? _____
3. How do the costophrenic angles compare? _____
4. Putting the history and x-rays together, the likely diagnosis is: _____
5. What accounts for the right mid-lung densities? _____

■◆■ CASE 8

1. The heart is bigger.
2. The pulmonary vessels are bigger and slightly less sharp.
3. There is fluid in the right costophrenic angle.
4. The patient is in congestive heart failure.
5. Fluid trapped in the major and minor fissures (pseudotumors). Fig. Q–8B shows the markedly thickened fissures.

"One day my father took me aside and left me there." John Vernor
"She got her good looks from her father. He's a plastic surgeon." Anonymous

■◆■

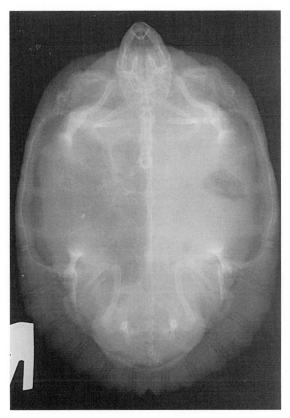

Figure Q–9

■◆■ CASE 9 ────────────────────────────────

HISTORY: "Swimming Lopsided And Looks Ill"

1. The _____ lung is consolidated.

2. This is an [alveolar/interstitial] pattern.

3. The patient swam _____ side down because _____.

4. The patient is a _____.

■◆■ CASE 9

1. Left (compare with normally aerated right lung).
2. Alveolar; the left lung is airless (water density).
3. Left; the left lung is heavier than the right lung.
4. *Trachemys scripta*—terrapin (turtle).

Dr. Timothy T. Klostermeier (a former resident of Dr. Felson) nursed the sick turtle back to health with daily subcutaneous shots of tetracycline for two weeks (Radiology 1996;199:58, with permission).

This case validates the "Purple Cow" theory of education. If you understand "purple" and you understand "cow," you will recognize a purple cow the first time you see one.

■◆■

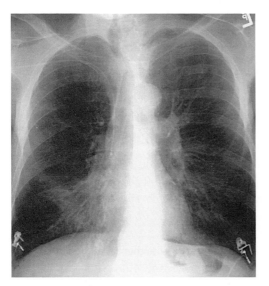

Figure Q–10A

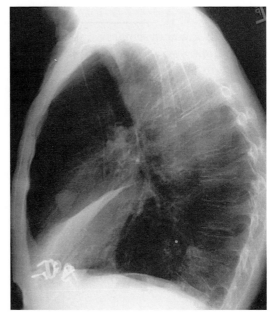

Figure Q–10B

■◆■ CASE 10

HISTORY: Smoker, With Cough For Three Months. Has A Known Goiter. There Are Four Potentially Important Radiographic Findings On These Films. This Is One Tough Case:

1. Years of smoking have caused what generalized lung problem? _____ Give four signs that lead you to that diagnosis. _____

2. A. On a frontal view, there is an alveolar infiltrate causing a silhouette sign of the _____.

   B. The silhouette sign and the lateral radiograph localize the disease to the _____ lobe.

3. The lateral view shows what additional focal lung problem? _____ Now localize it on the PA (if you can). _____

4. How does the goiter appear on the x-ray?_____

5. Combine the history and x-ray findings in 1, 2, and 3 to come to a unifying diagnosis. _____

■◆■ CASE 10

1. COPD (emphysema)
   Diaphragms are flat and low.
   Retrosternal clear space is increased.   ↑'d AP Diameter
   Upper lobe markings are sparse (bullae).
   Lung is hyperlucent.
2. A. right heart border
   B. right middle; note the atelectasis
3. A lung nodule is visible just above the collapsed right middle lobe. On the PA film, it is hiding lateral to the left atrial border, just beneath the left hilar vessels.
4. The cervical trachea is displaced to the right and narrowed. The cervical trachea is above the clavicles (feel it on yourself). An enlarged thyroid is the most frequent mass in this area.
5. The patient has COPD. A carcinoma obstructs the right middle lobe bronchus (not seen), causing atelectasis. There is a metastasis or a second tumor in the lingula. There is an incidental goiter (by history).

"It's not over 'til it's over." Lawrence A. Berra
"It's over." Lawrence R. Goodman, M.D.

■◆■

Index

Note: Page numbers in *italics* refer to illustrations.